MEDICAL ETHICS AND THE FUTURE OF HEALTHCARE

Edited by
Kenneth Kearon and Fergus O'Ferrall

Medical Ethics and the Future of Healthcare

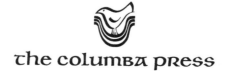

the columba press

First published in 2000 by
the columba press
55A Spruce Avenue, Stillorgan Industrial Park,
Blackrock, Co Dublin

Cover by Bill Bolger
Cover picture: *Anatomical Study* by John Hogan,
by permission of The National Gallery of Ireland.
Origination by The Columba Press
Printed in Ireland by Colour Books Ltd, Dublin

ISBN 1 85607 269 X

Contents

The Contributors

Professor James Childress is Kyle Professor of Religious Studies and Professor of Medical Education at the University of Virginia, USA.

Professor Walter Prendiville is Consultant Gynaecologist at The Adelaide and Meath Hospital, Dublin, Incorporating The National Children's Hospital, Tallaght and The Coombe Women's Hospital, Ireland.

Ms Verena Tschudin is editor of *Nursing Ethics: An International Journal for Healthcare Professionals.*

Dr Marianne Arndt is a lecturer in the Department of Nursing and Mid-wifery, University of Sterling, Scotland.

Dr Denis A. Cusack is Professor of Legal Medicine, University College, Dublin, Ireland.

Professor Marcus Webb is Professor of Psychiatry, Trinity College, Dublin, and Consultant Psychiatrist, St Patrick's and St James's Hospital, Dublin, Ireland.

Dr Patrick Hanafin is Lecturer in Law, University of Sussex, England.

Dr Sheila Greene is Senior Lecturer in Psychology, Department of Psychology, Trinity College, Dublin, Ireland.

Dr Fergus O'Ferrall is Director of The Adelaide Hospital Society.

Rev Canon Kenneth Kearon is Director of The Irish School of Ecumenics.

General Introduction

The Adelaide Hospital Society organised the major public lecture series in February and March 1999 on 'Medical Ethics and the Future of Healthcare' to facilitate better public understanding of the complex issues now confronting citizens and carers in healthcare. The contributions of the distinguished international and national lecturers were received by the public audience so well that the Society is pleased to be associated with Columba Press in making them available in a permanent way to a much wider audience.

As a voluntary charitable organisation dedicated to the advancement of medicine and nursing and to citizen choice in a pluralist healthcare service, the Adelaide Hospital Society provides an independent means for authoritative and considered contributions to health policy issues and concerns in the years ahead. This book is intended to assist public debate and discussion by the citizens of the Republic, so that they have the opportunity to shape their healthcare services in the twenty-first century.

Dr Fergus O'Ferrall
Director
The Adelaide Hospital Society

Introduction

In the world of television serials, hospital dramas have usurped the place formerly held by police dramas as preferred late night viewing. It isn't difficult to see why. Drama, tragedy, human interest, and life and death situations are part and parcel of modern hospital life, with each patient bringing his or her life story, needs, wants, hopes and fears into the hospital situation. Medical, nursing, and administrative staff have their own lives too and this can't but influence the way they work. An ideal context for a TV producer or scriptwriter in search of material for a new series.

The story line doesn't have to be too fanciful, for a modern hospital isn't all that different from a TV script. People are what nursing and medicine are all about, and that means that assessments of people, judgements about situations, advice and recommendations are being made continually. Rights and responsibilities, trust and concern, characterise the relationships between nurse, doctor, and patient.

In an ideal world judgements would be based on facts, rights and duties clearly set down for every eventuality, and advice determined by unambiguous experience, but medicine's concern with people means that this can never be the case. Every situation is different – feelings and emotions are as influential as facts and experience. It is in this complex world that ethics has increased in importance in recent years. Medical ethics is one of the oldest disciplines, dating at least as far back as Hippocrates in the third century BC. This tradition rooted in his famous *Oath* has served the world of medicine very well over the centuries.

Bioethics, on the other hand, is a very recent discipline (the term 'bioethics' only came into use in the early 1970s). It arose out of the questions generated by medical advances in the 1960s and 1970s when organ transplantation, kidney dialysis and life support systems became available with all their attendant ethical questions, with which we are so familiar today. These developments didn't reveal traditional medical ethical principles to be mistaken – instead, the sheer complexity of the questions raised meant that practitioners and those with clinical responsibility sought help in understanding the nature of the questions they were facing and how apparently conflicting principles might be balanced and resolved.

Thus was born the modern discipline of bioethics, which has been defined as 'the application of ethics to the biological sciences, medical health care, and related areas as well as the public policies directed towards them.' (*New Dictionary of Christian Ethics*, p. 61) It is an interdisciplinary subject, involving members of the nursing, medical and paramedical professions together with administrators, lawyers, and ethicists working together to ensure that rights, responsibilities, and, above all, the dignity of the patients and staff are respected and honoured both in the principles governing medical care, and the way sensitive and sometimes controversial issues are handled.

This approach determined the shape of the lecture series. The first half provides an overview of the issues. Professor James Childress takes the reader into the heart of the current situation, showing that bioethics emerges from a dialogue between principles and function, where reflection and concrete situations shape principles as well as principles shaping function.

This approach is reflected in the next three lectures, examining 'Ethical Issues in Women's Health', 'Ethics and Holistic Care', and 'Ethical Consideration in the Allocation of Resources in Healthcare'. Years of clinical experience infuse Walter Prendiville's approach to issues in women's health, and, in particular, his concern to see the number of abortions reduced. 'Holistic care', argues Verena Tschudin, begins with a genuine listening to the patient and her story; and Marianne Arndt's concepts of compassion, community, co-operation, and communications are essential values. Healthcare doesn't just happen. Administrators need to recognise the importance of these values and to reinforce the links to the structures of healthcare.

The second half of the series addressed four areas where concern for the patient as person generates controversial treatment. 'Issues in Patient's Autonomy and Consent' frequently appear in court cases. Denis Cusack guides us through the up-to-date situation in that area. The same issues reappear in Marcus Webb's lecture, 'Ethics in Psychiatry'. Few in Ireland could have been unaware of the controversy surrounding the Ward of Court case (often referred to as the 'Right to Die' Case). Patrick Hanafin puts this case in the context of a much wider international debate. Finally, Sheila Greene looks at the very topical and controversial issue of genetics and its impact on the person.

In conclusion, the editors wish to record their appreciation of the work of Ms Hyo Jung Kim, whose work in preparing this volume for publication was invaluable. They would also like to acknowledge the contribution of Ms Joan FitzPatrick, former Principal of the Adelaide School of Nursing, in devising this series.

Kenneth Kearon

CHAPTER ONE

Bioethics on the Brink of a New Millennium

James F. Childress

Introduction

Medical ethics often refers to ethics for physicians, parallel to ethics for other healthcare professionals, such as nurses. Not only did physicians develop their own codes of ethical conduct over centuries – as did nurses and other healthcare professionals as their professions evolved – but religious communities also promulgated rules for physicians, nurses and others. In view of these long-standing traditions of ethical guidance in medicine and healthcare, what is new and or distinctive about 'bioethics' or 'biomedical ethics' other than the terms?

Bioethics or biomedical ethics is broader than medical ethics or nursing ethics, and it extends beyond particular religious communities. It emerged in the late 1960s and early 1970s as part of society's efforts to deal with the moral perplexities occasioned by new medical technologies that could prolong life far beyond previous expectations, transplant organs from one person to another, detect certain fetal defects *in utero,* offer new reproductive possibilities, and the like. Bioethics involves an interdisciplinary and interprofessional approach to ethical issues in the life sciences, medicine, and healthcare.

My work in bioethics started in 1970 in my second year of teaching in religious ethics at the University of Virginia when I participated in an interdisciplinary and interprofessional faculty-student seminar on artificial and transplanted organs, with close attention to various medical, ethical, and legal issues. Even though I didn't realise it at the time, I had found my vocation, not only because of the excitement I experienced in genuine interdisciplinary and interprofessional exploration of difficult moral problems, but also because the issues were both challenging and important. Still, for several years, I resisted concentrating on bioethics because I was convinced that it was a temporary fad. In light of my dismal record in prognostication, I'm sure you'll properly discount any predictions I make about the future of bioethics.

It is difficult, if not impossible, to give a satisfactory overview of bioethics, which is my assigned task, because, even though this field is relatively new, it covers numerous topics – for instance, the second edition of the *Encyclopaedia of Bioethics*, published in 1995, consists of five long volumes. Instead I will offer some reflections about how we might do bioethics in the new millennium – these reflections will combine some thoughts about method with an analysis of moral issues in a few selected areas. Then I will close with some suggestions about how in the twenty-first century to hold together, in some tension, disparate elements in bioethics.

Moral Dilemmas, Quandaries, and Conflicts
Moral dilemmas, quandaries, and conflicts, as Stanley Hauerwas has stressed, don't simply exist out there in the world, like mud puddles we step into or walls we bump into. Rather they are created by our moral principles and values, by what we affirm as morally important. As a character in Tom Stoppard's play *Professional Foul* notes, 'There would be no moral dilemmas if moral principles worked in straight lines and never crossed each other.' Unfortunately moral principles do cross each other, in the context of the life sciences, medicine, and healthcare, as well as in other arenas of life.

This point really came home to me during a trip to the People's Republic of China about twenty years ago. Our delegation, mostly from the USA, Canada, and Germany, consisted of clinicians, philosophers, theologians, and others who were interested in how Chinese health professionals and policymakers approached problems in bioethics. We often asked them how they handled some of our 'problems,' such as an adult refusing life-sustaining treatment against the recommendations of physicians and family members. Most often our hosts responded: 'That's not a problem here. It doesn't exist here.' That response generally reflected China's different stage of technological development in comparison with western countries – at that time China lacked some of the biomedical technologies that were already widely used in the West.

Sometimes, however, that response – 'It's not a problem here. It doesn't exist here' – reflected different principles or values, or at least different interpretations and rankings of principles and values. In particular, our Chinese hosts were puzzled by our constant reference to individuals, their rights of self-determination, privacy, and the like. There is, for instance, no Chinese word for privacy, and yet, especially in the United States, 'privacy' has been appealed to in legal cases involving contraception, abortion, and termination of life-sustaining treatments.

If, in what our Chinese hosts insisted would be a rare occurrence, an adult were to refuse life-sustaining treatment against the objections of professional and familial caregivers, that person would simply be 'persuaded' to change his mind, just as family members reluctant to donate organs of a dead relative might be persuaded to change their mind or a family exceeding the recommended limit on the number of children might be persuaded to have an abortion. To those of us with ears attuned to more individualistic values, 'persuasion by talking' – the Chinese expression – seemed at times to verge on coercion, manipulation, intimidation, undue influence, and the like. However, our Chinese hosts did not view these situations and conflicts as 'moral problems' because their communitarian values easily trumped individualistic values. The latter generally did not provide enough counterweight to create 'moral problems.'

What is experienced as a 'moral problem,' then, and how it is resolved, will depend on the moral principles and values that individuals, professionals, and societies affirm. Those moral principles and values, whatever they are, set the stage for moral problems and conflicts and their possible resolution. We could, of course, eliminate some moral dilemmas, quandaries, and conflicts if we could reduce the number, weight, or strength of our moral principles – but in doing so we might sacrifice much that is essential to our conception of ourselves and our place in the universe.

Moral Principles

I will present a case that involves, to some degree or another, a wide range of moral principles that, many argue, are relevant to various issues in bioethics.

For the last three years a five-year-old girl has suffered from progressive renal failure as a result of glomerulonephritis. She was not doing well on chronic renal dialysis and the staff proposed transplantation after determining that there was 'a clear possibility' that a transplanted kidney would not undergo the same disease process. The parents accepted this proposal. It was clear from tissue typing that the patient would be difficult to match. Her two siblings, ages two and four, were too young to be organ donors. Her mother was not histocompatible, but her father was quite compatible. When the nephrologist met with the father and informed him of the test results, as well as the uncertain prognosis for his daughter even with a kidney transplant, the father decided not to donate one of his kidneys to his daughter. He gave several reasons for his decision: in addition to the uncertain prognosis for his daughter, his daughter had already undergone a great deal of suffering, a cadaver kidney might still become available, and he lacked the courage to donate one of his kidneys. However, he was afraid that if the family knew the truth they would blame him for allowing his daughter to die and then the family itself would be wrecked. Therefore, he asked the physician to tell the members of the family that he was not histocompatible, when in fact he was. The physician did not feel comfortable about carrying out this request, but he finally agreed to tell the man's wife that her husband could not donate a kidney 'for medical reasons'. (This case is drawn from Melvin D. Levine, Lee Scott, and William J. Curran, 'Ethics Rounds in a Children's Medical Centre ...' *Paediatrics* 60 (August 1977): 205.)

The physician felt uncomfortable in carrying out the father's request because of what he experienced as a moral dilemma. Appropriate responses to such situations often require close scrutiny of the relevant moral principles, what they mean and how much weight they have, in order to determine what ought to be done, all things considered. In this case the physician had to attend to a several moral considerations such as truthfulness, not lying, acting in the daughter's interest, confidentiality, protecting the father, and preserving the family.

In the fourth edition of *Principles of Biomedical Ethics* (1994) Tom Beauchamp and I use this case to discuss types of ethical theory; here I want to use it for another purpose: I want to use it to introduce some fundamental moral principles and show how they can and should shape the way we approach such a case:

(1) *Do not harm others*. This principle of nonmaleficence, as it is sometimes called, is central in the Hippocratic tradition of medical ethics in the maxim 'first of all or at least do no harm' *(primum non-nocere)*, which is not, however, part of the Hippocratic Oath. This fundamental principle generates some immediate problems in this case, because removal of a kidney from a healthy living person is intended primarily to benefit someone else, even though the donor may derive some moral or spiritual benefits from the donation. Thus, it is an atypical procedure. Even though over twenty donors have died in the USA, the risks of kidney donation are viewed as relatively low – that is, there is a low probability that a major harm, such as death, will occur. Donating a kidney usually doesn't change the donor's risk assessment for purposes of life insurance.

Furthermore, the physician in this case had to consider the possibility, emphasised by the father, that telling the family that the father could donate but didn't want to do so would 'wreck the family,' thus producing serious harm.

(2) *Benefit others*. In line with what is sometimes call the principle of beneficence, the father has a duty to act to benefit his dying daughter, and yet, because of the uncertainties in this case, it may be difficult to say that he has a duty actually to donate one

of his kidneys. The physician has a duty to try to benefit several people, including the dying girl, her father, and the family. And yet their various goods may conflict.

(3) *Maximise benefits; minimise risks; and produce a net balance of benefit over harms, burdens, and costs.* In such a case, in line with the principle of utility or proportionality, the physician may have to decide which course of action would produce the greatest balance of good over harm. It would be difficult, in this case, to say that the physician ought to try to persuade or even force the father to donate – the probability of a successful transplant does not appear to be high enough to warrant such an action.

(4) *Distribute benefits and burdens justly.* A principle of justice supports the professional judgement that the other children, ages two and four, are too young to serve as sources of a kidney – it would be unfair to impose the burden and risk of kidney removal on one of them in order to benefit someone else.

(5) *Respect persons and their autonomous choices.* The inability of the young patient's two siblings to give voluntary, informed consent counts against using them as sources of a kidney, even though in the USA families sometimes have the legal right to make such a decision (perhaps on the problematic ground that the child serving as the source of the kidney also benefits in having a sibling survive or in providing such a gift). The father's unwillingness to donate also raises the question whether it is ever justifiable to coerce someone to donate a kidney (or any other biological tissue). In this case the father's refusal was heeded.

(6) *Speak truthfully.* Even though the physician did not feel comfortable in saying that the father was not histocompatible – that would have been a lie – he was willing to say that 'for medical reasons' the father should not donate a kidney, perhaps because, in his judgement, 'psychological' reluctance to undergo elective surgery is medically relevant and thus constitutes a 'medical reason.' Nevertheless, the physician's statement to the family about 'medical reasons' would succeed only because he could expect the family to understand those reasons as biological or physical. If the wife asked, 'What medical reasons?' the

physician would be forced to answer truthfully or lie. Of course, out of conscience, he could simply refuse to be an instrument of the man's deception and let him explain the situation to his wife, either truthfully or falsely.

(7) *Act faithfully, keep promises, etc.* Perhaps the nephrologist was caught in a conflict of interest or loyalty because of his involvement with all the parties – we may need different physicians as advocates for donors and for recipients, rather than putting one physician in such a conflict of interest or loyalty. The question also arises whether the father was neglecting his duty of loyalty and faithfulness in abandoning his daughter, that is, by starting the tests and then backing out when it became clear that he and he alone could help her. In addition, the father's participation in acts that brought his daughter into the world engendered certain expectations, but it may be difficult to specify those in detail.

(8) *Respect privacy and confidentiality.* Perhaps the physician decided to say 'for medical reasons,' not because he believed disclosure would wreck the family – a consequentialist consideration – but because he believed that the duty of confidentiality outweighed the duty of disclosure to the family, specifically the spouse, in this case. Such an argument might take this form: in agreeing to undergo the tests, the father entered into a relationship of confidentiality with the physician, who then needed the father's permission to disclose this information to others.

There is a need for what might be called 'preventive ethics' – to avoid such a dilemma, quandary, or conflict – by making appropriate prior arrangements. More specifically, the physician in advance could have reached an agreement, or at least a solid understanding, with the family and its individual members about how such information would be handled.

This case indicates the relevance to bioethics of a wide range of moral principles. Even if there is a wide consensus that these principles are all relevant, several important disagreements may remain. First, there might be disagreement about the foundations of these principles – are they grounded in reason, in revelation, in social convention, etc? Second, there might be disagreement about how to interpret these principles, especially how to explicate their meaning, range, and scope. Here again fundamental theological and philosophical convictions may be important. Third, there might be disagreement about which principles should have priority if they come into conflict – for example, should either confidentiality or beneficence outweigh truthful disclosure in this case?

I will briefly focus on the second and third types of disagreement, which involve, on the one hand, specifying principles and, on the other hand, assigning them weights. Rather than approaching these types of disagreement abstractly or theoretically, I will explore them in the context of two contemporary controversies – one at the end of life and one at the beginning of life. One is long-standing, while one is new, but they are similar in that both controversies reflect scientific and medical achievements and both will persist well into the next century.

Specifying and Balancing Principles:
The Debate about Physician-Assisted Suicide
Clearly the principle of nonmaleficence can be further specified – it would rule out inflicting specific harms, such as death, and often creating the risk of such harms. One important specification of this principle appears in the rule: Do not directly kill an innocent human being. This moral rule would prohibit killing patients or assisting them in killing themselves by committing suicide. This prohibition has long been emphasised in medical and nursing ethics for various reasons, including the distrust that medical killing would generate. Not directly killing innocent persons is a fundamental moral rule that protects even patients who are suffering and dying.

A firm moral consensus developed over time in religious traditions and in the medical and healthcare professions: even though it is not morally justifiable to kill patients or to help them kill themselves, it is morally justifiable to let them die under some circumstances. Physicians and other healthcare professionals may, under some circumstances and within some limits, with-hold or withdraw some life-prolonging treatment, treatment that is considered extraordinary or heroic, so that patients may die, but they may not kill patients; they may relieve pain and suffering even though the drugs they provide may hasten death, but they may not kill patients or assist them in killing themselves. This consensus, which reflects one possible way to balance several moral principles, such as nonmaleficence, beneficence, respect for autonomy, and justice, has also been embedded in the law. But it is now under attack – the bright line between letting die and killing no longer seems so clear and compelling to many people.

The challenges to such long-standing professional, social, and legal rules often invoke different interpretations of these principles, especially respect for personal autonomy and benefi-cence, frequently expressed in the language of care and compas-sion, in the wake of a remarkable set of changes in dying over the course of this century. In the USA at mid-century, fifty per cent of the deaths that occurred each year occurred at home, but that figure declined to less than twenty per cent within thirty years, as deaths increasingly occurred in institutions, mainly hospitals and nursing homes. People live longer and die mainly from chronic degenerative diseases often diagnosed two or three years earlier. Not only is the process of dying longer, but dying also often occurs part by part, frequently leaving patients unable to express their wishes. Technologies, administered by strangers, can prolong dying, often at fantastic costs. It is no wonder then that many fear the process of dying more than death itself even though they may have little confidence in life after death.

This situation, accompanied by a new public willingness to talk about dying which was formerly a taboo subject, led to vig-orous efforts to extricate patients from the clutches of a techno-logically-driven system of medical care that appeared to threaten overtreatment at every turn. In the USA, the 'neon light' case that heralded so much change occurred 25 years ago – the Karen

Ann Quinlan case. Many other cases followed, as did legislation, such as natural death acts, primarily to apply the principles of respect for personal autonomy, for example, through advance directives to cover periods of incompetence, and beneficence/ nonmaleficence.

A number of patients and their families feel that it is not enough to let patients die by withholding or withdrawing treatments, or even to hasten death by medications intended to relieve pain and suffering. They want more – they want killing or at least assistance in self-killing. Some patients find their suffering too great, their dying too long, their control too limited, and they want to commit suicide with assistance, or they want others to kill them, rather than merely letting them die. They bemoan what they view as an undignified or undesirable death. And in a pluralistic society we have as many conceptions of a good death as we do of a good life.

Assisted suicide and some forms of euthanasia, or mercy killing, are very close. *The main difference is who performs the final act.* In assisted suicide, the one who dies performs the final act of killing, albeit with considerable assistance from others. In voluntary, active euthanasia, or mercy killing, someone other than the one who dies performs the final act, even though it is done at the request or with the consent of the one who dies. It is voluntary, not non-voluntary (without the person's consent) or involuntary (against the person's wishes). It is active, rather than merely passive. Recent debates in the US have focused on physician-assisted suicide rather than voluntary, active euthanasia – however, Dr Jack Kevorkian crossed the line to voluntary, active euthanasia in one of his recent cases.

The following case illustrates the moral concerns that challenge the traditional prohibition of physician-assisted suicide. Dr Timothy E. Quill, an internist in Rochester, NY, reported that he had helped a forty-five-year-old female patient, whom he had known well for eight years, commit suicide by providing her with a prescription for barbiturates and information on how to use them to commit suicide. The patient, Diane, had experienced several major personal and professional problems, including alcoholism, depression, and vaginal cancer, when she was diagnosed with acute myelomonocrytic leukaemia. This illness causes death in a short period of time if untreated but can be cured twenty-five percent of the time through major, extensive, and costly chemotherapy, and other treatments.

Diane decided, after discussions with her husband and college-age son, that she didn't want to undergo the treatments, but preferred instead to live her remaining days outside the hospital without chemotherapy, partly because she didn't want to suffer pain, loss of control over her body, and side effects from the treatment she was convinced would be unsuccessful. Her interest in maintaining control of her self and her dignity also left her unsatisfied with the prospect of comfort care toward the end of her life. 'When the time came,' Dr Quill said, 'Diane wanted to take her life in the least painful way possible. Knowing of her desire for independence and her decision to stay in control, I thought this request made perfect sense.' Furthermore, in various writings, Dr Quill has stressed the physician's responsibility not to abandon patients – an expression of the duty of fidelity – as well as to treat them compassionately and respectfully.

Whether we consider Dr Quill's act ethically justifiable or not, that particular judgement does not necessarily indicate what a society's laws and policies ought to be. In assisting his patient in committing suicide, Dr Quill put himself at legal and professional risk, because of the legal rules and professional norms against physician-assisted suicide, even though in fact he was not prosecuted or disciplined. Many argue that these legal rules and professional norms should be maintained, even if they are not always enforced, because they protect patients by providing a strong warning to potential agents of 'mercy.' Others argue for a regulatory approach that would bring the practice of physician-assisted suicide into the open and then limit the number and kinds of cases and set conditions for assistance. Some critics of this regulatory approach, which has been implemented in Oregon (and in a different way in the Netherlands), contend that it will alter the medical ethos and societal trust over the long run by legitimating medicine's involvement in killing; that its limits and conditions will not be maintained over time; that it will become an easy, efficient way to respect autonomy and act compassionately, thereby diverting efforts to relieve pain and suffering through appropriate palliative care, as employed in the hospice movement; and that some patients will feel coerced by this option. Such critics often stress further that it is a terrible mistake for the society to accept physician-assisted suicide when adequate healthcare, including palliative care, is not widely available, especially in the USA, which lacks universal access to healthcare. A few other critics find regulation too restrictive and would allow physicians and patients to work out their own arrangements about physician-assisted suicide, subject only to the general societal and legal constraints that govern physician-patient interactions. However, the main debate is between the first two positions – prohibition and regulation.

Specifying and Balancing Principles:
The Debate about Cloning Human Beings
Until 1997 I had never included the topic of human cloning in my bioethics courses. I concentrated instead on 'realistic possibilities' – the only 'science fiction' I assigned was Aldous Huxley's *Brave New World,* mainly to show how many of his 'prophetic' judgements had come true. I didn't focus on 'mere possibilities,' such as cloning humans. And yet with the announcement by Ian Wilmut's team of Dolly's birth, through the process of somatic cell nuclear transfer cloning, my picture of the future changed – suddenly, human cloning had emerged as a realistic prospect.

The immediate public response to the prospect of producing a child by cloning was outrage and fear – everywhere cries were heard, 'repugnant,' 'revolting,' and 'offensive'. Even Ian Wilmut found this prospect 'offensive'. But the immediate question was how the society should respond through its laws and policies, whether through a ban (either temporary or permanent), regulation, or permission – in short the same policy options that arise for physician-assisted suicide.

In the USA, the Clinton administration immediately declared a ban on the use of federal funds for research to clone humans, called for a similar voluntary moratorium in the private arena, and asked the National Bioethics Advisory Commission (NBAC), on which I serve along with seventeen others, to prepare a report and make recommendations within ninety days on appropriate public policies responses to the prospect of cloning a human being.

NBAC's report, *Cloning Human Beings* (June, 1997), recommended continuing the moratorium on the use of federal funds for research related to human cloning to create children and continuing the voluntary moratorium in the private arena. In addition, NBAC recommended federal legislation to prohibit, at least for the time being, somatic cell nuclear transfer to create children. NBAC rested its recommendations, at least in part, on the following argument: 'at this time it is morally unacceptable for anyone ... to attempt to create a child using somatic cell nuclear transfer cloning ... because current scientific information indicates that this technique is not safe to use in humans at this time.'

Some critics charge that NBAC, a 'bioethics' commission, failed because it based its recommendations on a scientific argument about safety rather than on an ethical argument. That charge reflects an inadequate understanding of ethics. More accurately, in light of the available scientific evidence, NBAC reached a moral conclusion, based in part on the ethical obligation not to harm, or impose serious risks of harm on, potential children. Safety is a fundamental ethical consideration. It is not merely a scientific consideration, even though it obviously requires scientific evidence. Any procedure that creates a substantial risk of harm to children is morally problematic.

Some commissioners were apparently also convinced by other ethical arguments concerning potential psychosocial harms to children (e.g., to their autonomy and independence), wrongs to children created through cloning (e.g., objectification and commodification), threats to the family, etc. Others, who found the physical safety argument compelling and sufficient, also noted that a temporary ban would give the society time to think through the whole range of ethical issues in order to determine whether cloning human beings to create children should be permitted, regulated, or prohibited, once the safety barriers have been overcome.

The following is an actual case of deliberate conception of a child that I will later modify to raise questions about whether in similar circumstances producing a child by cloning would be ethically justifiable. In July 1989, a middle-aged couple from a Los Angeles suburb deliberately conceived a child in an effort to save the life of their teenage daughter who was dying of cancer. The couple (Abe and Mary Ayala) had learned two years earlier that their daughter, Anissa, was suffering from leukaemia and needed a bone marrow transplant to survive, but no one in the family was a compatible potential donor and no unrelated donor had been found.

They had only a slim chance of conceiving a child at all; Abe had to undergo an operation to reverse a vasectomy performed sixteen years earlier, and Mary was forty-two years old. Even if they could conceive there was only a 25 per cent chance of a bone marrow match. The baby (Marissa), born on April 3, 1990, was a good match, some of her bone marrow was latter transplanted to Anissa, and the transplant was successful. A few years later Marissa was the flower girl at her sister Anissa's wedding.

If a family faced the same situation as the Ayala family, if their daughter's leukaemia resulted from environmental causes, rather than genetic factors, and if human cloning could be safely used to create a child who would be a perfect bone marrow match for the dying daughter, would that be ethically acceptable? And should such cloning be permitted, regulated, or prohibited? In a society, such as the USA, that fails adequately to regulate various reproductive technologies, it may be difficult to prohibit or even to regulate human cloning. Perhaps as a result, in contrast to several other countries, the USA has not yet prohibited human cloning to create children, even temporarily, despite NBAC's recommendation. Nevertheless, if human cloning were safe for the children created this way, the scenario above might plausibly qualify for an exception under a regulatory scheme, if all the rights and interests of the child were truly protected.

Tensions in Bioethics on the Eve of the twenty-first Century
In conclusion, I would stress that bioethics in the twenty-first century will need to hold together several elements that are frequently in tension.

First, as these two case studies suggest, ethical judgements may well and often should vary depending on whether they are directed at acts, at practices, or at public policies. All of these are important, and none should be neglected. However, a judgement about one of these does not necessarily dictate a judgement about the others. For instance, holding that a particular act, such as assisted suicide or cloning a human being, is morally wrong does not necessarily imply that it ought to be legally prohibited. And holding that one of these acts is morally right, at least under some circumstances, does not necessarily imply that a practice is right, much less that an ethically acceptable public policy would permit or at most regulate such acts, rather than prohibiting them altogether. Applying moral principles to particular cases, to practices, and to public policies may lead to different conclusions.

Second, as these case studies also indicate, no single moral principle can be taken as the sole determinant of judgements about acts, practices, or public policies. For instance, the temptation in a liberal society is to assign priority to the principle of respect for personal autonomy, which, taken by itself, could support permissive public policies toward physician-assisted suicide and human cloning. The critical task for bioethics is to determine how to specify and to weight the full range of relevant moral principles in the context of concrete acts, practices, and policies.

Indeed, one important substantive undertaking for bioethics, in whatever problems it confronts, is to discern the proper balance between individual and community. One major charge frequently directed at much western bioethics is that it is too individualistic. Some argue that we need a principle of community, beyond what might be implicit in the principles I identified, or at least that we need to reinterpret those principles in a communitarian way – for example, respecting persons as social and thus as members of particular communities, religious and otherwise. This point is well taken, but it needs to be addressed cautiously. We do not need another 'ism' – communitarianism to replace individualism. What we need instead is to discern, in response to different issues and problems, the proper balance between the claims of individuals and the claims of communities.

No doubt what is perceived as the proper balance between individuals and communities will shift over time, as well as the proper balance among the various principles I identified. In their book *Tragic Choices* (1978), Guido Calabresi and Philip Bobbitt argued, with specific reference to policies to allocate scarce life-saving medical resources, that societies make tragic choices, sometimes invisibly, sometimes visibly. What makes a choice tragic is that some principle or value is compromised or even sacrificed in order to protect other principles or values when it is not possible to realise all of them simultaneously in the same situation. However, Calabresi and Bobbitt note that the pendulum swings over time, and that a society can sometimes reaffirm a principle or value it neglected earlier by giving it additional or special attention over time. It is thus important to think about the proper balance over time, without using time, or the possibility of future redress, as an excuse to neglect principles or values that could in fact be protected at the moment if we exercised greater imagination and creativity.

Third, even though I have focused on moral reasoning in this paper, it is crucial not to separate or oppose reason and imagination, particularly when considering future possibilities. Moral imagination, according to Patricia Werhane, *Moral Imagination and Management Decision-Making* (1999), includes 'the awareness of various dimensions of a particular context as well as its operative framework and narratives. Moral imagination entails the ability to understand that context or set of activities from a number of different perspectives, the actualising of new possibilities that are not context-dependent, and the instigation of the process of evaluating those possibilities from a moral point of view.' Moral 'problems', as I have emphasised, are not given but are structured by our perspectives, including our principles and values. Hence, it is important to keep in view a wide range of possible ways to structure problems.

Another important exercise of moral imagination is to discern in routine, ordinary established patterns of conduct ethical issues that have been obscured or neglected. The case studies I examined involve dramatic moral conflicts, but through the exercise of moral imagination we can discern ethical issues that pervade the life sciences, medicine, and healthcare even though they do not rise to the level of dramatic moral conflicts.

Agents exercising their moral imagination can also discern features of new situations or new cases that are morally relevant in part by perceiving their similarities to and differences from established precedents – this is a process of analogical reasoning that has been emphasised by the casuists. In addition to moral imagination, agents need various traits of character and dispositions to properly interpret principles and situations and also to discharge obligations and realise ideals.

Fourth, bioethics is not merely a matter of 'applying' moral principles, such as the ones I have stressed. The metaphor of application is too narrow, and it neglects or distorts much that is important in bioethics. In addition to deficiencies already noted – for example, the need for interpretation through specification and weighting and the need for imagination – the term 'applied' suggests that bioethics resolves problems instead of setting them, that its solves puzzles instead of providing perspectives, that it answers rather than raises questions, and that it begins from theory rather than from lived experience. The term 'applied' implies a limited technical or mechanical model of bioethics.

It also ignores the numerous theoretical controversies in bioethics, and it neglects the way bioethics may help to resolve or recast some theoretical controversies. At the very least, the metaphor of application may need to be supplemented by various other metaphors for the task of practical ethics, including bioethics, which may involve theory, conceptual analysis, diagnosis, etc., all of which go beyond the kind of technical role that the engineering model of 'applied' ethics tends to emphasise. Some other metaphors are drawn from ancient religious roles, such as prophet or scribe. Yet another metaphor is 'conversation,' which is prominent in approaches to bioethics that emphasise interpretation, hermeneutics, and narratives.

Fifth, no doubt the 'professionalisation' of bioethics is important, particularly as this field becomes more rigorous and more accountable. Nevertheless, bioethics is too important to be left to professional bioethicists, whether philosophers or theologians or others. In my judgement, bioethics is necessarily interdisciplinary and interprofessional. The professional theologian or philosopher can contribute to this discourse mainly by explicating traditions of moral reflection in order to illuminate current debates. Others can contribute in other ways. However, no single professional group has more moral insight or wisdom than any other – the participation of all the relevant professional groups, along with broad public participation, is indispensable to good bioethics. This model of broad participation requires attention to a wide range of religious and philosophical perspectives, for example, in the debate about cloning humans.

In this regard, it is also important for bioethics to hold together, frequently in tension, insider and outsider perspectives – or, in different language, proximity and distance. Both proximity and distance are needed – proximity to the felt problems in science, medicine, and healthcare, and distance that allows a critical perspective. Both are indispensable in adequately understanding and structuring 'moral problems'. How those in the medical trenches or on the medical firing lines construe their experiences is exceedingly important, but critical distance may also be valuable in setting the problems to be resolved.

Finally, bioethics must be sometimes be prophetic – 'Woe unto you …' Many of us may be seduced by proximity to power – the power of decision-makers whether in the clinical setting or in shaping public policy. We may become very good at what Daniel Callahan calls 'regulatory bioethics,' while, in the process, neglecting to speak in a prophetic voice, even when morally appropriate or imperative, for fear that we will no longer be invited to the table for discourse about bioethical issues. To contribute in the twenty-first century, bioethics must include prophetic as well as regulatory approaches, just as it must hold together in some tension the other elements identified in this conclusion.

CHAPTER TWO

Ethical Issues in Women's Health

Walter Prendiville

In this paper, I have been asked to address the title 'Ethical Issues in Women's Health'. There are many problems in addressing this subject. The first of these is that I am not an ethicist. I am a working clinician who sees patients every day. I have no expertise or training in the discipline of ethics, unlike today's graduates from some of our more enlightened medical schools.

However, I believe that I do know that some things are right and that some things are wrong. Indeed each and every one of us believes this whether they are doctor or priest, technician or teacher, manufacturer or labourer. To some degree we would all consider ourselves ethicists.

At least we all have opinions, and in Ireland we have little difficulty in airing them. Bar room ethicists abound and amateur philosophers are ten a penny. Political parties and divisions spring up all over the place. They say that if three British people met on a desert island they would form a queue, whereas if three Irish people met on a desert island they would form a political party! We like to think of ourselves as intellectuals who have each thoroughly considered every philosophical issue.

My own profession is not perfect in this regard. No two doctors will agree on every aspect of care for every patient in every circumstance. This does not inevitably lead to the oft quoted 'Doctors differ and patients die'. This is because there are many ways of expertly managing a number of conditions. For some of these there is good evidence that the best method is known but for many others it is not.

For example, in these islands the routine method of managing the third stage of labour (when the afterbirth is delivered) is to give an oxytocic drug to help the uterus contract and to then gently but firmly pull on the umbilical cord in order to deliver the placenta. I recently asked a friend of mine who is a Professor of Obstetrics in France how the third stage was managed in his country. He assured me that it was quite standard and followed by saying that the *accoucheur* simply waits for the placenta to be delivered and that hands off policy prevailed throughout the country. Indeed he declared that one of the few ways for a medical student to guarantee a career outside medicine was to advocate pulling the umbilical cord. Further, in France it is absolutely routine that every antenatal examination is associated with a vaginal examination. In these islands a vaginal examination would be most uncommon until labour or at least the very end of pregnancy.

These are huge differences in practice. In these circumstances someone must be right and someone must be wrong. But tradition has dictated different fundamental practice in two large neighbouring countries. Different right and different wrong.

However, the medical profession is rapidly becoming convinced that we should operate according to the best evidence rather than according to what we were taught or what a particular textbook said or even what our own particular experience has suggested. In this I believe that we are probably ahead of the other professions.

However, convincing let alone proven evidence is only available for a relatively small number of circumstances. Diseases and medical advances change rapidly. It is not always possible for evidence-based research to keep up with these changes. Often we have to rely on less reliable means of assessing the best way in which to look after our patients. However, for 99% of doctors, I believe that the essential principle of doing what one believes is best for the patient rules absolutely. Whilst I might not agree with the actions or advice of every doctor I come across, I respect his or her right to do so providing that person is acting according to this principle.

There are, of course, other principles that come into play

when assessing a doctor's performance, such as being up to certain standards of the day, having sufficient knowledge to be able to give informed advice and being able to communicate appropriately. For the purposes of this discourse, however, they need not interfere with the basic tenet of this argument.

And this is all very well for the prescription of antibiotics for a bacterial infection, for the surgical correction of a specific physical abnormality or even the vaccination of a population against, say, tuberculosis. It becomes more complex, ethically speaking, when the intervention or advice pertains to social or personal circumstances which affect the way normal people live. Then a doctor may be accused of interfering with nature, or society, in a manner not fitting with the accepted expectations of some members of that society.

An example of this might be fluoridation of our water supply or the prescription of high doses of morphine for terminally ill patients who are in pain. There are probably no finer examples of this to be found than those in the realm of reproduction. In this sphere we are all truly experts and the same principles appear to prevail. Each of us believes that we have the common good at heart, that we know what's best for our society and the individuals within it and that the evidence for our stance is unequivocal, convincing and supported by the ultimate higher authority.

There are a number of circumstances when we can interfere in the natural history of reproduction. First we may try to improve a person's chances of conceiving by using pharmacological or surgical techniques. A number of eventualities may arise which will pose difficult ethical questions for the couple, the doctor and the society in which they live. Even if it improves the chance of success, is it ethical to produce several embryos that may never see the light of day? What is one to do with these embryos? Should they be frozen or discarded? Should they all be re-implanted even it this increases the risk of miscarriage? Should we try to clone a human being? If so who should it be? Mother Teresa? Michelle Smith? Bill Clinton?

These are difficult questions that have been the subject of intense scrutiny by a number of national and international bodies at medical and non-medical levels. These questions are difficult, demanding and important subjects. However they affect a relatively small number of people. They are not within the brief of this talk

Rather I would prefer to discuss the question of preventing pregnancy. Here we have a number of ethical issues that affect nearly every person in this and every other country. I contend that there are very few couples in Irish society today who do not wish to control their fertility at some stage during their reproductive life.

Birth Control: The Prevention of Unwanted Pregnancy
There are several dimensions to birth control. There is the global issue of overpopulation. Do we already have too many people in the world? Is it reasonable to try to control the world's, or a part of the world's, population at this point in time? What is wrong with having as many people as possible?

But these are subjects that tend to interest a relatively small proportion of people. Most of us are less concerned with what goes on outside Ireland than that which goes on within. And within Ireland we are more concerned about what goes on within our own sphere of influence than without. We are more interested in what goes on in our own personal life than in other people, at least for most of the time!

And our own reproduction is intensely interesting to each of us. To reproduce has profound implications for the way in which we live our lives. It is a serious responsibility for both parents and changes us utterly. To reproduce is a wonderful thing. It is an amazing thing and in the very great majority of cases a truly beautiful and rewarding experience. But the circumstances must be right for it to be so. Very few, if any, of us would choose to conceive at the extremes of reproductive life (i.e. as young teenagers or in our late forties). Very few of us would choose to conceive if we were in poor health or extreme circumstances of poverty or during a famine or during a major episode of turmoil in our lives.

And nature does not get it right every time. Indeed nature does not get it right even most of the time, especially during the first third of pregnancy. Perhaps surprisingly, the majority of conceptions miscarry. Most do so before a woman has realised that she could be pregnant. And even after a pregnancy is clinically recognised and after a pregnancy test has become positive, somewhere between fifteen and twenty per cent of pregnancies will spontaneously miscarry. Occasionally one of these will be because of the pregnancy implanting in the tube rather than in the womb. This produces a life-threatening event that will usually warrant surgical intervention to end the pregnancy in order to prevent catastrophic and life threatening haemorrhage.

But there is little profit in blaming nature for these events. And for the great majority of pregnancies which do make it past the first trimester a live and healthy baby will ensue.

So what and when are the precise interventions that are available to couples to prevent unwanted pregnancies? They may be conveniently divided into three categories:

Contraception (Pre and Post Fertilisation)

Sterilisation

Termination of Pregnancy

Each of these poses an ethical dilemma, or to put it another way, may produce an argument in Ireland. It's perhaps fair to say that, in other Western European countries, the arguments surrounding both pre fertilisation contraception and sterilisation have had their day and that these methods of birth control are broadly accepted as reasonable interventions at both a personal and societal level. Raaran Gillon, in an editorial in the *Journal of Medical Ethics* in 1998 entitled 'Eugenics, Contraception, Abortion, and Ethics', argued that '… religious considerations apart it is difficult to see how voluntary birth control (where a couple do not wish to have a baby) can be regarded as morally objectionable'. But we live in Ireland and this is not so. Relatively recently we had a situation whereby the apparently

harmless activity of selling condoms became a national and legislative conundrum of ridiculous dimensions. I don't need to re-
hearse the history of contraception in Ireland because time does
not allow but surely no one would disagree that it has been a
longstanding political and legislative mess.

And why is this? It seems to me that there are essentially two
opposing camps addressing the problem of unwanted pregnancy.
These are the secular and the religious. The secular view is that
an individual or couple have the right to decide when and how
many children they wish to have by choice rather than chance. It
appears to me that the very great majority of women and men
that I meet take that view and put this creed in practice in their
lives. Yet for some of the established religious traditions, notably
the Judeo-Christian ones, they seem to be at odds with their
flocks on this fundamental ethical issue.

The Religious View on Reproduction, Women, Contraception,
Abortion and Sterilisation
This is a complex subject about which much has been written
both from within and without the different churches. Also a
church's view is a dynamic thing and has changed in many
ways throughout the last two decades, which is surely a good
thing. The church with which I am most familiar is the Irish
Roman Catholic Church. Its view is quite clear. Pope John Paul
II reaffirmed that the procreative function in which man and
women collaborate with God in the propagation of the human
species, according to the plans of his transcendental economy, is
sacred. Perhaps I'm wrong but it also seems to me that the Irish
Roman Catholic Church has embraced this philosophy more en-
thusiastically than other European churches.

The [Roman] Catholic Church condemns any direct attempt
against the life of the innocent, against the life of the human being
who is developing in the womb of the mother. Furthermore *in*
utero, the embryo with a defect 'should not lose the prerogative
of human beings, he or she should be given the respect due to
any patient'. The same statement is reaffirmed in *Evangelium*

vitae. Finally the Roman Catholic Church considers that human life begins at conception as opposed to implantation.

This view about the collaboration of man and woman with God in attempts to conceive appear entirely reasonable if sexuality were a purely procreative phenomenon. But many within and without the Roman Catholic Church accept that this is not so and that sexuality is a positive, normal and beneficial part of a mature bonding relationship between a man and a woman which is completely independent to the question of reproduction. It is also widely acknowledged, again by many within the Roman Catholic Church, that a couple should not always strive to produce children. In these circumstances what are a couple to do? They have the following choices before them.

Contraception (Pre-Fertilisation)
1. Abstinence based contraceptive options:
Rhythm, Temperature and Mucus recognition systems with or without the help of biomedical technology are all based on the same basic premise. This is that it is possible to reliably recognise the so-called fertile period by identifying ovulation. By avoiding intercourse during and around this time a couple would be able to have sex without fear of conception during the remainder of the cycle. All of these methods therefore rely, for their effectiveness, upon partial or total abstinence during the apparent fertile period. For some reason that I don't fully understand, these abstinence-based methods have been described as 'natural' rather than 'artificial'.

On the other hand, the advantages of these methods are that they have the blessing of the Roman Catholic Church and that they don't require any medical interventions. The disadvantages of these methods are that they are all, and they are by far, the least effective of the contraceptive options available. This does not in my view mean that they should be dismissed out of hand. If a couple is fully informed about the pregnancy rates associated with these methods then they are perfectly entitled to use them and they may reasonably expect their doctor to be able to competently and non-directionally inform and advise them as to how the methods work. For some couples a relatively high pregnancy rate is an acceptable price to pay when balanced against the perceived disadvantages.

2. Barrier methods:

Condoms, diaphragms, female condoms, and caps are all essentially means of trying to physically introduce a barrier between the sperm and the upper female genital tract. They are associated with pregnancy rates (pearl indices) of about 3-5 pregnancies per hundred women per year. Condoms have the additional advantage of affording some protection against sexually transmitted diseases but all the barrier methods have the disadvantage of being perceived by many to be interfering with sex either before or during coitus.

3. Oral contraception:

The pill has been the most tested, the most prescribed and the most powerful of influences throughout the world during the last thirty years. Time does not allow for a comprehensive review of the pros and cons of different pills that are available, but there would be a reasonably consensus view in the medical fraternity that the combined oral contraceptive pill is a safe, effective and reliable model of contraception for the great majority of women. For those with particular predisposition to thromboemoblic disease the progesterone only pill (or injection) is an attractive alternative but has a slightly higher pregnancy rate (roughly similar to the intrauterine contraceptive device). One of the infrequently quoted benefits of the combined pill is that for women who have ever used it for a year there is a forty per cent lifetime reduction in the risk of ovarian cancer.

Post-Fertilisation Contraception
1. The Intrauterine contraceptive device:

The coil or IUCD probably works primarily by preventing implantation of the fertilised egg in the uterine wall. It is associated with a relatively good pearl index of about one to two pregnancies per hundred women per year. It has several advantages and several disadvantages. The most obvious disadvantage is that there is a small risk of pelvic inflammatory disease or PID and this risk is greater in younger women. The risk of PID in one large study in London's Margaret Pyke Centre revealed a tenfold increase in risk for women under 20 when compared with women over 30. The coil is therefore largely reserved for women over 30 who have finished their family. The other difficulty with the coil is that it probably works post-fertilisation and pre-implantation.

2. The Intrauterine system or MIRENA:
The MIRENA is an intrauterine device that incorporates a hormone delivery system. In other words it is a coil that also releases a small amount of progesterone into the uterine cavity on a daily basis over five years. These two combined mean that the intrauterine system has an exceptionally low pregnancy rate. An added bonus is that for most women their menstruation disappears. It is for this reason that the MIRENA is as popular as a means of treating heavy periods as it is as a contraceptive. However the device is a relatively large IUCD and therefore is usually reserved for women who have had children. It is particularly popular in Northern Europe and is growing in popularity in the UK. It is a very real alternative to sterilisation and has the advantage (over female sterilisation) of not requiring a general anaesthetic.

3. Post-coital contraception:
There are several methods of post coital contraception but the two most popular are the oral combined oestrogen 1 progesterone pills taken as 100megms twice 12 hours apart and the IUCD. Oral post coital contraception is perhaps more commonly known as the morning after pill which is a little unfortunate because it means that some women believe that the medication must be taken within 12 hours to be effective and this is not so.

The method is effective if taken within 72 hours. The IUCD also works if inserted within 5 days of unprotected intercourse because, as we mentioned above, the coil's method of action is primarily to prevent implantation of the fertilised egg.

Ethical Issues Concerning Contraception

1.i. Pre-fertilisation contraception: Is it morally right?

Whilst there are some, there are probably few people in our country who now fervently believe that it is wrong for a couple to plan their family size and timing according to their circumstances. Once this is accepted, much of the argument about contraception evaporates. Some people will argue that the free availability of contraceptive advice and information will lead to uncontrolled promiscuity. But the number of people holding this view is dwindling. Furthermore, the evident advantages to an individual couple of being able to prevent an unwanted pregnancy far outweigh any theoretical change in societal norms. Even our health boards now support the concept of providing contraceptive advice to all those who require it.

1.ii. Pre-fertilisation contraception: Is natural more ethically sound than artificial?

A fundamental difference between the artificial and natural methods is that the former attempts to prevent conception effectively whilst at the same time interfering as little as possible with the sexuality of intercourse, whereas the latter is firmly based on avoiding the sexual component of intercourse and accepting a relatively flawed contraceptive effect. Natural methods of contraception are all based on avoiding intercourse either temporarily or completely (sometimes known as the Rhythm and Blues). One could be forgiven for thinking that the obsession with natural method morality had more to do with particular attitudes to sexuality than with fertility control.

Again, there is the purely religious view that contraception can only be morally acceptable if it is based upon the concept of sexual abstinence. The fact those natural methods are, relatively speaking, the least effective has led most couples to vote with their feet and adopt the more effective methods.

2.i. Post-fertilisation contraception: Is this abortion?

There appear to be three different ethical standpoints when discussing the question of post-fertilisation contraception. Firstly, there is the view that life begins at fertilisation and that the fertilised egg is a full person from that moment onwards. Secondly, there is the view that conception starts with fertilisation but that it is a process that is only completed after implantation.

Finally there is the view that personhood, or humanity, is not conferred upon the fertilised egg until some time later in pregnancy. Embryologists, philosophers, and theologians will disagree about when this time is but many would agree that it is not until after implantation. In considering this issue, the following may be helpful:

a) Over half of all pre-implanted blastocysts will fail to impact and will be lost with the next menstrual flow. No alteration in menstrual flow or timing will be noticed. Is it right to equate these cells with a human being when nature is so unconcerned with their fate?

b) The blastocyst faces certain destruction unless it can prevent the next menstruation. It is only after implantation that the hormone human chorionic gonadotrophin enters the bloodstream thereby maintaining the corpus luteum, thereby preventing the next menstruation.

c) After implantation, the embryo becomes able to dictate the hormonal and other circumstances whereby it has a reasonable chance of surviving to term and delivery.

While the absolute view of humanity beginning with fertilisation has an immediately and simple attractiveness it does not sit comfortably with nature's appreciation of the status of the pre-implanted blastocyst. Indeed, it could be argued that the blastocyst has a near equivalence to the egg or the sperm in that they are all potential until conception has been completed at implantation. John Guillebaud argues these issues cogently and states that because prior to implantation there is no carriage and therefore pre-implantation interventions can rightly be considered contraceptive rather than 'procurers of miscarriage'.

To many these arguments are akin to how many angels can dance on the head of a pin. Do they matter? Do people consider them important issues? It would appear that in Ireland these issues are not widely thought of as impediments to practice. The IUCD is relatively popular and post-coital contraception is more popular here than almost anywhere else in Europe. This probably reflects other difficulties with contraceptive availability, accessibility and acceptability, but more of that later.

Sterilisation

There is little that needs to be said about sterilisation from an ethical point of view. Providing, of course, that one accepts that the decision can only be taken after fully informed counselling. There seems little to argue about apart from religious concerns surrounding contraception in general. Counselling must include consideration of the failure rate, irreversibility, and complications of the technique, the fact that it can be performed under local or general anaesthetic for male or female and a full discussion of the alternative methods available. There is, however, a very real ethical issue for healthcare providers. If one does not allow sterilisation to be performed in a hospital that cares for women, then there will be a greater number of unwanted pregnancies than would otherwise occur. Furthermore, and I remember this well from my junior days as a trainee obstetrician, where sterilisation is not allowed in a hospital the threshold for performing caesarean hysterectomy falls, as will the number of women requesting such operations. Having said this, for most people the ethical issues around the question of sterilisation are of historical interest only.

Termination of Pregnancy or Abortion

Is abortion ever right? Nobody has a monopoly to being right about issues of conscience and personal morality. I do not pretend to know the answers to all the questions about abortion. But I am sure that we, as a society, will benefit from discussing these very complex issues in public without rancour or acrimony and with the common ambition that prevention is better than cure. I hope that we are mature enough to do so. From my own perspective, the following points may be helpful:

1. The very great majority of Irish women who have a termination of pregnancy do so for social or personal reasons that have nothing to do with medical, psychiatric, or psychological risk to the mother.

2. For the very great majority of women who have a termination of pregnancy, there is a very, very small risk of long term psychological trauma or sequelae.

3. There are definitely medical conditions whereby a pregnancy constitutes a profound risk of death. These conditions are rare, but when they occur the women who have them should be made very aware that pregnancy constitutes a very real threat to their lives. They deserve such informed and non-directional counselling both before and during early pregnancy when a termination may well prevent them from dying. Examples of such conditions would include Eisenmenger's Syndrome and any condition associated with pulmonary hypertension. The evidence to support this is widely acknowledged by specialists working in areas where these conditions occur. They do occur and women do die from the extra physiological burden of pregnancy. But they are not common circumstances. In Ireland, we might expect to witness such cases once every decade, but they are becoming more common. There are also other conditions where termination of pregnancy may be considered an indirect intervention, performed in order to treat the disease (for example, cervical and other forms of cancers), but in the full knowledge that the treatment will abort the foetus.

4. Irish women are having terminations of pregnancy at a similar rate to many other countries in Europe, but are seriously disadvantaged by the lack of both pre- and post-termination of pregnancy (TOP) counselling facilities here in Ireland.

Furthermore, because of the lack of pre- and post-TOP medical care, more Irish women are likely to suffer from the complications of TOP, especially because of the lack of a routine post-TOP follow-up scan and assessment one to two weeks post-op. There is much that one could say about the rights and wrongs of abortion and those who are interested and who have not yet immutably and irrevocably formed their opinions are referred to Ronald Dworkin's excellent book on the subject. There appear to be two essential ethical standpoints that are diametrically opposed to each other. On the one hand, the anti-abortionists would maintain that life is sacred and that it starts with fertilisation. On the other hand, the supporters of abortion would maintain that life is sacred and that no one has the right to interfere in a person's life, particularly in relation to the control of her reproduction.

The anti-abortionists would argue that the mother does not have the right to take the life of the conceptus, foetus, embryo, or 'unborn child'. The supporters of abortion or pro-choice camp would argue that the State or authority does not have the right to insist that a mother carries a pregnancy which she does not want or can not accommodate socially, personally, medically or physically. Both positions, whilst being diametrically opposed to each other, are also quite similar. They are each absolutist both in their essential contention and in their dismissal of the opposing argument. Also, both sides derive their moral justification from the standpoint of having profound respect for human life. The pro-choice camp wishes to see total respect for the mother and the anti-abortionist wish to see total respect for the (foetus) pregnancy.

Yet, for most people the situation is really quite different. The subject, which is so often discussed in black and white terms, is actually very grey. To be more precise, most people do not see the issue in black and white terms. Most people have different views about abortion according to the circumstances under consideration. I don't just mean that a person might have a different view if they found themselves the subject of interest. That is human nature.

And there is a spectrum of opinion concerning how to deal with the issue for each and every case that presents. For example, whilst many people will be very anti abortion on demand, there is perhaps considerable support for women in particularly tragic circumstances. Recent highly publicised cases such as the x or c cases support this concept. Take the case of a woman carrying a foetus with a medical condition that is incompatible with life (for example, anencephaly). Such a woman would, I contend, be likely to meet with a sympathetic public and, indeed, usually a sympathetic doctor. Finally, a woman with a medical condition that threatens her life would also be likely to meet with broadly sympathetic public support if she requested a termination of pregnancy. She would probably also meet with a supportive response from many doctors, who at this time, would of course have to look outside the State if they wanted to help their patient in this way.

But in many ways, these are side issues. They are real issues for the very few women who are unfortunate enough to be in one of these situations and I don't want to diminish the gravity of any particular case. But they are indeed rare circumstances. And rare circumstances make bad law. To legislate according to the rare case, almost by definition, ignores the reality of the common circumstance. In Ireland, 99% of women who have crisis pregnancies and who opt to travel abroad for a termination of pregnancy do not have a medical condition or a congenitally abnormal foetus. They simply do not want to have the pregnancy continue. It is about the common circumstance that we should spend most of the time deliberating and legislating.

The issue of abortion highlights the other classic example of how an ethical question should not usually be considered in black or white terms, as a yes or no dichotomy. The spectrum of gestational age (how far the pregnancy has progressed) has a huge influence in this regard. It is true that some philosophers will view gestational age as being irrelevant when considering the rights and wrongs of abortion but for most doctors and couples, this is simply not the case. To put it another way, it can be argued that life is life and therefore any attempt to terminate a pregnancy is wrong. However, very few people view the few cells of a pre-implantation conceptus in the same light as a six-month foetus. By the time a foetus has reached six months it has been acknowledged as a human being and has had its personhood recognised. This is not so for the three-day-old pre-implantation fertilised egg.

At a practical level this is best exemplified by the use of post coital contraception. This form of post fertilisation very early contraception is widely viewed as being morally acceptable and indeed a positive phenomenon. Whereas termination of pregnancy in the second or third trimesters of pregnancy, particularly in the absence of a serious medical condition of the mother or a serious foetal abnormality, is widely considered by both doctors and society as essentially wrong.

There are perhaps two explanations for this phenomenon. Some people might say that as human beings we are actually more influenced by the aesthetics of abortion than by the ethics; that we can accommodate the simple prescription of a post coital pill but not the aesthetic reality of a mid-trimester abortion. The other view would be that, for the very early pregnancy that involves a few unrecognisable cells, the pregnancy is not perceived as being a human being and that it has not yet reached human status.

No ethicist, philosopher, gynaecologist, or theologian can tell anyone what is right and what is wrong in relation to the difficult question of abortion. For many, it will be a case of obeying the decrees of their religion. For others, it will be peer or parental influences that dictate the ethical view. For each of us, it is not easy. For every stance there are likely to be seriously opposing opinions.

To close I would like to highlight those aspects surrounding abortion upon which there is virtual unanimity of agreement. Too many Irish women are having abortions. It is not in women's interests that this continues. It is not good for doctors. It is not good for the government. It is not good for our religious advisors. It is not good for our society. It is not good for anyone.

And yet our society seems paralysed to do anything about it. Both sides of the debate agree that it would be preferable if we didn't have so many abortions. Both sides of the debate seem to agree that these women need caring for. But to an outsider it might reasonably be assumed that no one wishes to take responsibility for instituting strategies to address these two needs.

So, what are our ethical responsibilities in relation to abortion amongst women in Ireland? With regards to the attempt to reduce the number of women having an abortion, we probably all have a responsibility. With regards to caring for women who have a crisis pregnancy, the responsibility lies with healthcare decision-makers and providers.

Ethical responsibility for those who wish to witness a reduction in the rate of abortion in Irish women
I cannot think of any one who would not wish to see the current rate of over 5,000 women per year reduced. If we as a society are to realise a reduction in this number, then we will have to implement some strategies designed to achieve this ambition. It is not going to change on its own. Clearly the current *laissez faire* attitude of all of us (and I include my own profession and speciality) has not worked and we have been implementing this approach for some time.

There are two approaches to the problem and, unfortunately, they are philosophically quite different. The first is to provide a comprehensive programme of sexual and reproductive education for our children so that they may be prepared for sexuality and to then provide an effective family planning service that is truly available, accessible, and user friendly. The second is to persuade our population to change the current sexual mores, so that the risk of an unwanted pregnancy disappears or is profoundly reduced.

My own view is unimportant, but either way, and even if we decide to do both at the same time, what is clear is that we need to start very soon.

CHAPTER THREE

Ethics and Holistic Care

Verena Tschudin

I have a very good friend, Pat, who finds the most wonderful postcards. One of these shows a steep roof by moonlight, and a person standing on a rope stretching from the roof. The person is standing on the far end of the rope and while one foot is on the rope, the other foot seems to step out into nowhere. What's more, this does not seem to be a dream, but reality. I want to use this picture as the basis for what I want to develop. It will set the tone for this paper; that is, I want to be somewhat speculative, looking to the personal; and into corners that may be a little dark and perhaps not always visible to everybody yet.

Holistic Care

Let me start with holistic care. All good work starts with a definition, and so I looked up the word 'holistic' in my *Chambers Dictionary*.[1] There I saw that the word 'holism' was coined by General Smuts. When I looked up Jan Christian Smuts (1870-1950),[2] I was reminded that he was a South African politician, field marshal, lawyer, and Prime Minister. He was also a segregationist, voting in favour of legislation that took away black rights and land ownership. It doesn't mean that those who understand the theory of something can also put it into practice. A further search for a definition led me to the *New Dictionary of Medical Ethics*[3] that states that 'holistic is used to describe an approach to medicine that takes account of the whole person, rather than focusing on solely medical aspects'. Arguably, this is an essential feature of good medical practice in any system.

The American Holistic Nurses' Association is a little more specific. They say 'that nurses have the unique ability to provide services that facilitate wholeness. The concepts of holistic nursing are based on a broad and eclectic academic background, a sensitive balance between art and science, analytical and intuitive skills, and the opportunity to chose from a wide variety of modalities to promote the harmonious balance of human energy systems. The teaching/learning process enables nurses to assist people to assume personal responsibility for wellness. We believe that disease and distress can be viewed as opportunities for increased awareness of the interconnectedness of body, mind, and spirit.'[4] This seems to give an indication of what is actually involved in holistic care; let's see how it works.

I have heard practitioners of complementary therapies say, almost in despair, that people do not understand the underlying philosophy of these therapies. They treat them like they would treat orthodox medicine, i.e. when they have a headache they want a remedy that works and buy that, rather than see a headache in terms of the whole person and all that this may point to. Indeed, in the West, we are used to going to a doctor and telling her or him what is matter with us and a diagnosis will be established on that basis. In the East, people go to their doctor and say, 'Tell me what is the matter with me.' The answer may not be as easy as 'you are stressed, therefore you have a headache'. However, I want to use the word 'holistic' in a much broader sense than simply referring to certain therapies and systems of care.

Anyone who has ever had a series of tests is very well aware of the concept of holistic care by experiencing the lack of it. Someone examines your eyes, someone else your ears, a third person your stomach, a fourth is interested in your lungs, a different clinic in your skin, and the queue for blood tests is never ending. There could be something drastically wrong with your soul, your family, the energy field in which you live, or because of the kind of work you do, and nobody may know. Some of this must be happening to anybody suffering from those conditions we have today which are labelled as mysterious and for which no-one wants to take responsibility, such as M.E., 'Gulf syndrome', or organo-phosphate poisoning. If there is no clear answer, you might be labelled neurotic or obsessive. If so, you get sent to the psychiatrist and get yet another diagnosis. With so many possible specialities available, it is tempting to make them all work by referring patients and clients to as many of them as possible. This may make practitioners feel good because they have thought of them all and ticked off all the possibilities on a list, but is that 'holistic'?

Healthcare and medicine tend to concentrate on what is broken, diseased and not functioning. They see selectively and therefore in fragments. They see neatly, each bit fitting in with another. If there is something wrong in your head, there is a neurologist to deal with the head, or if you have cancer of the bowel, you see a gastro-intestinal oncologist. Each ailment is geared to a speciality, uniquely equipped with machines and statistics to get the best possible result for this particular diseased part. When the magic has reached its end, there is always palliative care, which means that we have an answer right up to the end. Is this holistic care?

There comes a point when more technology is only oppressive, and when more of what's wrong with you is destructive of what is actually working, right, good and whole. If we talk of holistic care, then we need to start from the positive, the good, the possible, and the whole.

That starting point, however, is not that easily grasped. When someone has a broken arm, surely it is more important to fix the arm than to spend valuable time on all the other limbs and systems that are working well. Maybe a healthy young man or woman falling off a ladder and breaking an arm does not need a great deal more attention from the health services than getting the arm fixed and into plaster and a little physiotherapy afterwards. But if this healthy young person is a professional violinist, she may not be able to continue her career. The broken arm is only just the tip of a very big iceberg reaching into the depth of the person and who and what she is, where and how she lives, and who and what supports her. We know this scenario, and this is not the place to elaborate on it. I simply want to mention it and point up the long and perhaps narrow road which holistic care is in comparison with the wide and short road of the healthcare system we know so well. I also want to point here to the way of thinking which is necessary if we start at the other end of care: when the person is at the centre, not what the person suffers from. Fixing a broken bone is easy and quick, but the consequences may be long – very long lasting – and still go on when the original problem no longer exists.

Holistic care in hospitals and the community is basically the same in theory, but in fact the problems encountered tend to be diametrically opposed. I will start by looking at a few facts about hospitals.

I have permission to tell you of a person whom I have long respected enormously. Michael Wilson is a doctor who for many years worked as a missionary in West Africa and when he returned to the UK worked as a GP. He became a priest and in this dual capacity worked for many years in pastoral theology. He wrote a number of books (the most famous is *Health is for People*[5]), constantly stressing that death is part of life and that we need to regain a respect for death. If we do not, our affluent nations will become bankrupted as we spend more and more money on unobtainable goals in healthcare. He stressed this in all he wrote, arguing that death is a friend, not an enemy. A few months ago I received a letter from him saying that he has a lump in his neck which is an aggressive lymphoma and he has decided not to have the chemotherapy that might be the only possible way to prolong his life by a few weeks. He writes in this letter: 'For the last thirty-five years I have written about health and death, living and dying, in books and articles, and spoken of these things in lectures. Now I must live what I stood for.' But he is doing this not as a kind of 'it's caught up with me now so I must be brave', but writing of an opportunity to make something positive of the experience. He sees all this as affecting not just himself but also his family, friends, neighbours, doctors, and church community. More than that, he sees it as a common journey – 'our' journey – which will affect many unknown people also. In this way, it is affecting your journey by me telling you about it. He is concerned that he is not using more of technology than he can square with his conscience. He quotes an earlier colleague of his whom said, 'A particularly nasty way of being greedy is to steal my brother's healthcare resources.' With his experience of work in West Africa, this is very poignant. Michael says, 'Please enhance my normality! A lump in my neck is not the centre of my universe.' He quotes Rilke: 'Do not seek answers, which cannot be given you because you would not be able to live them. And the point is to live everything. Live the questions now.'

Here is a person who tried all his working life to give holistic care and when it came to him, he found his experience of medical and hospital visits 'oppressive'. He found it 'stifling' that everybody concentrated on what was wrong with him rather than what was right. He needed to defend himself by appealing to his friends to keep him normal. He writes of a common journey, taking the rough with the smooth. He is lucky he can reason and write; plenty of other people could not.

In the community the conditions are different in that it tends to be the people with long-term conditions who are cared for, or those who need a 'finishing off' time after a spell in hospital. The problem there, at least in the UK – the scene which I am most familiar with – is more of how care (in the form of nurses, care attendants and equipment) actually gets given, that enough of it gets given, or the right quality. The 'care by postcode' trend can be very demeaning. Too often it seems that whatever you want these days – or more possibly need – has to be fought for. Clearly, technology is much easier to have and give than human resources and human care. Yet, without 'humanity' any kind of care, even technological, is pretty useless.

As you will have gathered by now it is extremely difficult to describe or be sure what holistic care is. I have concentrated on what it is not, and in that way pointed to the shortcomings. By its very nature, it is not possible to make a list of what holistic care may or can include. It depends on the persons concerned, the environment, and the conditions. This is not an excuse for not trying to explain it. If I had tried, I would have been sure to have left out the most important element for someone. However, having shown up some of the areas where it matters if the principles of holistic care are not applied, I hope I will have raised the issue enough to take it seriously. I want to leave the topic therefore at this point and turn to ethics, coming back to holistic care later.

Ethics

In 1986 I had my first book on ethics published,[6] and I started the preface with: 'Ethics is ... thousands of answers'. A reviewer pulled me up on this and said that this is nonsense; ethics is something very precise and possible to describe in a few principles. The more I tried to accept this, the more I had difficulties. To me, ethics is also in how one says 'Good Morning' to a patient or client, and how someone brushes passed you in the street as if you did not exist. It may be that these come under the heading of 'beneficence' or 'respect for the person' but this is such a wide concept that we can get lost in it. Ethics is something that affects everybody differently, therefore we cannot have just one, or even a few answers, but we need very many.

Ethics is necessarily related to 'good'. Thomasset makes the point that 'ethics expresses a wish, a fundamental desire for the accomplishment of being, and the aims of a life lived according to actions considered good.'[7] Morality, he says, 'is reserved for designating that group of norms, imperatives and interdictions which fall on the side of "obligation".' He sees ethics to be inspired by teleology, emphasising an orientation toward the good; and morality characterised by deontology and duty. An 'ethical aim has to pass through the filter of moral norms, in order to test its validity ... [that is] ... norms function as criteria of validity for all our ethical desires towards the good life.' The question is how we can access the 'ethical desire' and what gives meaning to action and ultimately to life.

An unusual stance is taken by Taels who writes of a narrow and a broad approach to ethics. He sees autonomy, as leading to a rationality that is narrow. More knowledge demands more knowledge while all the time leading us away from the actual ethical task. Today we have to be educated about 'world history, literature, politics, social and religious affairs … racism, employment, security, education, environment, and so forth'. In this task, we forget our own selves and direct, interpersonal relationships are removed from the ethical scene and discourse.[8] Since we cannot keep up with all these issues, we tend to flee 'the unbearable burden of global (political) responsibility into indifference or cynicism'.[9] The broad approach, on the other hand, is 'closely related to the complex of concrete day-to-day relations one has with oneself and one's environment'.[10] It demands a concrete ethical attitude that is based on 'thoroughness, honesty, a sense of justice, fidelity, and honouring one's word'.[11] Such attitudes have to be discovered and lived by individual persons in their own original way. It is in becoming self-aware that one becomes a 'concrete ethical being'. This means that becoming self-aware is a basic ethical duty. When we are self-aware, we have the ability to recognise real ethical needs and make real ethical decisions. When we are self-aware, we are able to distinguish between personal needs and common needs, personal desires and common desires. Rather than be cynical or indifferent, we are able to engage at a level which is realistic. Not only are we able to stand alone but also stand together, judge for ourselves and be responsible. On this analysis, the need – even the duty – to be and become self-aware seems to be the primary ethical duty. It is also the place where we start with what is good, right, functioning well, and whole.

In order to become self-aware we have to listen to ourselves and to others. We hear ourselves in telling our own story and we hear ourselves when we listen to others' stories. Listening seems absolutely fundamental. Knowledge is only useful if we can distil it into something that nourishes the person and in turn can be used for rightful action.

Health professionals must necessarily interact with patients and clients in whatever work they do, but do they hear what a person has to say? What story does the person have to tell? So that this can happen, the professional needs to be able to listen, and that means not just making the ears work, but have the capacity to listen with the whole person, heart, soul, mind and body. Professionals must be capable of being present. This is perhaps the biggest task for health professionals to achieve. For patients it represents the biggest obstacle they meet. For employers it represents time and money. Any nurse or doctor will tell you that they have not enough time for this sort of work. These are the points where ethics is met and touched upon, and becomes visible and recognisable.

Many years ago, I trained as a counsellor, and it was that which led me to ethics. Now I usually find that when I am with people for counselling I help them to work out the ethical problems in their life, and in my work on ethics I stress the basics of counselling, namely to listen. We need to listen to hear a story; we need to hear a story so that we can relate to a person. All of us – we may be clients, patients, professionals or whatever – can only make sense of life and any action by talking about it, telling someone about it. We have to express ourselves in order to be, become, and remain human.

Ethical listening is listening to the whole person and the whole story, not only selected parts. This takes time and effort. It is so much easier to ask a few pertinent questions and then be proud of reaching a diagnosis quickly. People are more than a diagnosis. They are more than an illness. The problem is that the story changes in the telling. One person may hear this aspect and another person another. The story grows and matures. The problem that many health professionals have is how much 'truth' someone ought to be given or can cope with. However, the problem is rather what is the truth at the moment because tomorrow it will be different anyway. In terms of holistic care, it means that whatever truth is available matters. It does not mean that it is quantifiable. It matters that whatever goes on between any two people, both can live with it and grow through it. If we apply this to others, we also need to hear this ourselves. Self-awareness comes not from being alone, but from being engaged with others. Our self-awareness grows in relationships.

Most of you are probably familiar with the work of Carl Rogers, at least with the three elements of counselling which he had established: genuineness or congruence, unconditional positive regard, and empathy.[12] These attitudes are basic to any real human interaction.

You know when you have met genuineness. It is there in the look and the body language. I think most of all it is there when you tell someone something good that happened to you and the other person is pleased with and for you, genuinely. Someone is genuine if what they think and say is the same thing.

Unconditional positive regard is a kind of steadiness. The humanity of the other is valued – full stop. Not just bits of a person are seen and acknowledged as good, acceptable or worthy of attention, but all of the person counts. It is possible to grow in this attitude with a person in the sense of the more you know, the more you respect the person.

Empathy is understanding and appreciating the feelings of another person and being able to communicate this to the other person. Empathy is supremely a two-way process. Sadly, we know it too often in its absence.

When we can be genuine, warm, and empathic with others and ourselves, we listen respectfully, ethically. When we listen in this way, we do not make any assumptions, either about people, diagnoses, treatments, outcomes, or possibilities. Making assumptions is giving people labels and making sure the labels stick. Nor should we impose values of health and illness on others that demand practically that they be followed, or else … This is a paternalism of a very pernicious kind. Ethics is about what is good and right, especially in relation to power. When we are able to accept other people as they are, and be with them as we are, then we do not need to make labels or impose our values. When we do that, we are equal with others and human with

others, and power does not play a big role. This, in my understanding, is what basic ethical listening is about and what leads
to ethical relationships.

The Implications of Caring Holistically

Let me then turn more specifically to ethics in holistic care and
to the implications of such care. Most of us who have been teaching ethics in healthcare settings find that starting with theories
and principles does not make sense to students. Healthcare professionals rarely find themselves in situations where they say,
'Ah, now this is an ethical dilemma, which principle is most relevant here?' Nurses and doctors find themselves with a person
or in a situation where something has to be done or said and
they do this on the basis of their conscience, what is 'right' at
that moment. If they are lucky, they will have the opportunity to
reflect on what they said afterwards with others, when principles and theories may be considered. If we have tried one approach to healthcare and have found it not working well, we
clearly need to find one that works better. From what I am saying, it is the way of relationships and relating.

By saying that stories have the power to be the decisive force,
I may be accused of advocating uncritical egoism. If you ask
anyone what he or she wants in the area of healthcare, and com-
ply with his or her wishes, you will ruin the system. Anyone
with kidney failure wants a transplant; anyone with a child who
has leukaemia will want all the treatments available. Anyone
with impotence wants Viagra. Anyone with multiple sclerosis
wants cannabis. Anyone who wants an injection to be put out of
his or her misery will get it. We have seen plenty of such stories
given wide treatment in the press and the pros and cons of the
arguments are well rehearsed.

We need to look at these scenarios a little more closely.
Maybe you remember the story of a child with leukaemia who
had treatment refused at a famous London hospital and whose
father then got treatment for her from a private sponsor. I felt at
the time, and actually said to one or two people, that I thought

the father could not come to terms with the child's possible death. I could only guess, from reading between the lines of what I read and heard. When the child died a few months later I heard on the radio something to the effect that the father could not bring himself to tell the child that she was dying and that he had pushed the treatment for her because of his needs. It seemed to me at the time such an obvious scenario and I wondered why nobody had helped the father to tell his story.

In *Nursing Ethics*, the journal that I edit, I have published more than one article relating stories of patients who were not granted their wishes and therefore died a rather painful death. The one that I have in mind is told by a nurse whose uncle James was admitted to the ward where she worked. James had a fairly severe left-sided hemiplegia due to an earlier stroke and it was thought that he now suffered from disseminated cancer of the prostate and was waiting for test results. James had told a cardiologist that he did not want to be resuscitated in case of a cardiac arrest, but that he wanted 'to go peacefully'. However, the cardiologist specifically instructed the nurse caring for him to disregard this. The next day, Christmas Day, James did indeed have a cardiac arrest in the shower and was resuscitated in the corridor, at length, because of complications. His niece came on to the scene as this was happening and so awful was the scene she did not recognise her uncle. He died the next day in the coronary care unit when his life support machine and inotropic infusion were stopped.[13] The man had said what he wanted but he was not heard.

Over Christmas, we had a few cases of children dying of meningitis. Someone who created a radio programme on this topic interviewed four different sets of parents who all told stories of going from GP to GP and hospital to hospital and still the child died. In each case, the parents said the same thing: 'They didn't listen.'

Patients and clients are not heard. They are either not given the chance to tell their story or their story is ignored. Why? The simple answers must lie in what I have already mentioned. We have not enough time to listen. We are afraid of what we might hear. We think we know better. In other words, we do not give holistic care.

To think that we know better must surely be the most basic infringements of human rights. When we make assumptions and impose our own values we declare ourselves superior, better, or simply different from others. We do this on the basis of professional competence and knowledge. Yet, what characterises a profession is not that it keeps its knowledge for itself, but that it shares it. When we keep knowledge to ourselves, we infringe professional ideals and rules. When we do not give holistic care and we do not act ethically, patients may be rightly entitled to complain and even sue the practitioners. This may have repercussions for the health service that we may only imagine.

When we are afraid of what we might hear, we show that we are not self-aware. If we think we may hear something with which we cannot cope, or which might give us offence, then we are not yet able to function as fully human beings. There is never a point at which we arrive and when we can say 'now I am self-aware' or 'now I have reached the necessary insights to be usefully human'. In order to be human we have to 'become' human. We can do this only in relation to others. If we want to be able to function as professionals in the caring field, we have to develop the genuineness, unconditional positive regard, and empathy I mentioned. Only in this way can we become 'unshockable', and this is one of the basic needs for holistic care. Holistic care demands that we are able to hear everything, see everything and think everything without labelling it as 'good' or 'bad' before we have heard all of it. We owe it to our clients and patients that we can be as human as possible.

If we take this implication seriously, then we look much further than simply medicine and nursing. It is a fact that we learn our morals and ethics as children. It is in school that we are taught how to reflect, think and reason. Therefore, it is in the education system that we need to learn how to listen to others and respect what we hear. Much more of this needs to be learned later also. The basic point here is that if we want to be holistically ethical, we need to have the kind of education and learning environment in which this is possible, starting with our basic schooling, and through professional education and in continuing learning and teaching. The programmes are there, but they need to reflect this particular need much more clearly. Only when we have a climate of care and support from the top down can we give holistic care from the bottom up.

When we do not have enough time to listen to a story, we are impoverishing ourselves and society. If we do not have time to listen, we may have to have time (and money) later for repeated admissions, bigger bills than necessary for drugs, more dependency, more ill-health and misery, more of that common journey which is existence rather than life, and more of heartache and mistrust of everything to do with healthcare. This affects us as individual practitioners, but it affects in particular the politicians and governments who have to allocate money. All the managers of 'human resources' know how difficult it is at the present time to get this right. Perhaps it is partly due to terminology. Are we simply a human resource? Maybe the word 'personnel' was not exactly right either, but when we do not deal with real people with names, it should not surprise us that we have problems. When we are dehumanised, we cannot give human services. No wonder then if we cannot and are not willing to give the most valuable thing we can give to others, namely our time.

Time and people mean resources again, and here we may be speaking directly of money. Rationalisation and cuts here and there have reduced the service to its bare bones almost everywhere. Everybody knows that bare bones cannot function alone. They need the flesh on them. Patients cannot get better if left alone. They need nurses and doctors to care for them. People are a health service's most costly resource in terms of finance. Maybe we should use the word 'costly' in its positive way: the most precious and dear in terms of human beings.

I expect that all of us have experienced the situation when we simply sat with someone, perhaps in silence, and something so profound happened in that time that the lives of both people have been affected, maybe in quite intangible ways, but you know it. Perhaps someone sat with you at a moment of crisis and was simply there for you. If holding a child, cuddling a frightened adult, or sitting with a dying person is never a waste of time, then how do we not recognise that in less dramatic situations such giving of time is also necessary? To spend twenty minutes now with a person may literally save us real money and time later. It is in such moments that we learn what is good, right, just and whole much more than what is broken, ill, or wrong. We start with what is positive. That is what holistic care is about in the first instance and to be aware of this is also ethical care.

It is very easy to see all this mainly in terms of economics and value for money and all those ideas like efficiency and effectiveness. In human terms, however, we cannot reduce everything to something that can be measured in pounds and pence. Life is more than a bottom line. We are often, however, in danger of forgetting this. When we do, we need to recall that perhaps we have left out the other 'e' word: ethics. To return to the argument I made earlier about ethics emphasising an orientation towards teleology and morality towards deontology, a further point needs to be made here. Thomasset points out that what is ethical will have had 'to pass through the filter of moral norms in order to test its validity'[14] and I understand this to mean that to act ethically we have to be aware morally. If politicians and managers ask us to act ethically but do not give us the possibility to act also morally, then we have a problem. If they ask us to give holistic care but do not enable us to be holistic people, then there is a dilemma.

Time is perhaps the most precious thing we can give to another person. When we give of our time, we give of ourselves at our deepest level. We make it clear to the other that 'you are important', 'you matter to me'. With this, we convey something so fundamental that it is the beginning and end of healing and restoring, that is, of all healthcare. If we do not have time, we cannot listen and we walk past humanity; our own and that of the other person.

Caring holistically involves time above all. It is not necessarily length of time that matters, but the quality of that time. Nurses are concerned about this more than anything else. Their care now has to be so carefully documented that they have time only for the documents, not for the care. The documents are needed for statistics, for league tables and for career prospects. It is very sad if in the process the humanity of it all gets lost. Hospitals are getting more and more to be places to avoid. Not only do patients come out more malnourished than when they went in, but they also come out humanly more damaged and degraded than when they went in. Yet, I also know that doctors, nurses and all concerned with patients do a terrific job, not because they can, but because they want to, and despite the system.

I would like therefore to ask, can we afford not to give ethically holistic care? Can we afford not to pay most attention to the stories we need to hear? Can we afford not to listen? Simply in terms of money – value for money – we cannot.

Giving ethically holistic care means first that we respect each other as equal partners of the human race. Even though equal, our needs are clearly different. Take the people whose stories I recounted. The father, whose story of his dying child was not heard, thereby put his child through an ordeal – simply in terms of human suffering – which might not have been necessary. It made good copy for the media, but I think they were probably the only people who profited from the story. I can only guess that now the father and mother of the child, the nurses, doctors, social workers and even the sponsor of the treatment for the child are all in some way damaged psychologically. They will all ask themselves how it is that no one took the time, dared to hear the story and was so sure they knew better. Similarly James, the old man who did not want to be resuscitated. Why was he not respected? The pain of all this even in terms of money is huge. The fall-out in terms of humanity is phenomenal. We cannot measure the guilt, mistrust, and feelings of incompetence, being let down and abused. At best, people can deal with them, given time. At worst, it may be two or three generations from now that their descendants can let go of some shadow that fell upon the family at that time.

I am firmly convinced that when we take time to listen to our clients and patients we do not hear only stories of 'I want' and impossible requests. I think that quite rightly, if heart transplants are held out as the cure-all, someone may want a heart transplant. Or someone may ask repeatedly for active euthanasia. Yet when we really listen, we may hear that a heart transplant is not actually the best option for a particular person, but it may be that a particular doctor puts this forward as an option because that doctor does not know how else to deal with the patient. Or that a person's request for that injection to end life is indeed the deeper request to be acknowledged. Too often, it is that health professionals cannot cope with suffering, and in an effort to make any situation 'alright', they distort what is happening. Van Hooft says that 'the key point about an authentic acceptance of suffering is that suffering is not made meaningful'.[15] Only when we can hear the other person express the meaninglessness of suffering, life, or whatever concerns them, and accept this, have we heard that person; only then have we truly listened. We cannot take the suffering away from someone else; we can only relieve it. What we can and surely must do is be ready to accept the other person. When we can listen, we will hear the real, the actual story, and that story may be about something different from what it may look like at first. I think that, like Michael Wilson, many more people will actually want to say 'no'. They will say that they don't need spare-part surgery. They don't want weeks of vomiting and feeling literally like death warmed up when it will not make any difference. I think also that many more doctors will actually be able to 'let go' of patients if they work in a climate where this is possible rather than always holding out the spurious hope of one more drug or treatment. When we can listen to someone's story, we may hear the meaning of her or his life rather more than the loud and often angry 'I want' or 'I need'.

The dilemma of scarce resources is part of all life and has always been. Since we live at a time when we know so much about world problems of employment, the environment, education, homelessness, etc., but feel incapacitated by these problems, we have to be able to set free our 'desires towards the good life'. We can only do this when we can be responsible and engaged, and we can only be that when we are treated with respect, honesty, justice, and truth. Holistic care therefore is first of all 'just' care, and I mean the word 'just' in the broadest sense of sharing what we have. When the professionals share with their clients what they have, the clients can share with the professionals what they have. Health professionals need to acknowledge that their clients and patients also have ethical desires towards the good life and need to be ethically engaged. Professionals, above all, need to enable such ethical action and responsibility. The implications of this, too, are that the climate has to be right for justice, truth, honesty, fidelity, and honouring one's word to be seen as good. Our whole society is concerned here. Yes, people have a right to complain and use the law when they are not treated, as they should be. Too often, however, we abuse our power and then it is very difficult to get back to truth and honesty. Society does not change such attitudes overnight, but in healthcare where an ethical principle of 'truth telling' has been conspicuously absent, we need to be concerned that we do our bit in this generation to put it in, perhaps for the first time since Hippocrates.

One way in which we can and must learn to do this is by being less tidy in our thinking and believing. Now we have a diagnosis, prognosis, and treatment. If it fits with what the book says, it is given a name and follows a known trajectory. But people are not like that. We may all have the same anatomic systems, but as unique individuals, these systems work individually. As professionals, we need to learn to live and work with ambiguity, uncertainty, and fuzzy edges. My knowledge of physics is not good enough to be precise, but I understand Chaos Theory not to be something indeterminate but rather something that works with astounding complexities. Taking indeterminacy and actually using it as the reality has then become the inherent feature of Quantum Theory.[16] When we can learn to work with the unpredictable and the indeterminate, we are more closely connected to human beings and human life than we are with exactness and with scientific precision.

When we can be more open and more uncertain in our dealings, we become more free and more joyful. We become more creative and imaginative. Too much healthcare now stifles our creativity. If Michael had such a job in being able to affirm his personality and humanity – and he is a doctor – then what chance do people have who are less knowledgeable and less articulate? When we are able to hear a person's story, we also hear their language and expressions and we can adapt our language to theirs. Then we do not speak down to them but with them. I am sure that for many professionals this is like stepping on to a rope stretching from a roof in the middle of the night. The only light is the moon, and even that is reflected light. Perhaps this is precisely what is needed.

Conclusion

We can only become increasingly ethical beings through the stories we make and tell of our lives. The saying goes of a man who said, 'I don't know what I think until I have said it.' Ethical principles only make sense when we can reflect on our stories and see what may have happened. In the moment, we have to consider what is happening, and that means an engagement with life itself and with the people in our lives. It means interacting and being open to what we may meet and meet it without judgement or assumptions.

The moral implications of this have to do with our willingness to be self-aware not only for our own good but also for the sake of others. Self-awareness is often painful and is basically a never-ending process. As professionals, we have a duty of continuing education. Self-awareness, self-assessment and self-challenge must be one such duty. When we give up the engagement with our own selves and our lives, we lose the right to be called professionals. Somewhere at the bottom of the moral implications of holistic care is that thorny question if we are and should be 'our brother's keeper'. The language bothers me in this phrase, and I would prefer to say that we are responsible to each other. As professionals, we certainly are responsible to our clients and patients.

The financial implications make it clear that with the rapid changes in health care as we experience them at this time, it becomes ever more important that holistic care is given. Technical and scientific care alone is far too expensive. It may have prolonged life – though that is questionable since environmental factors are likely to have played a bigger role – but it has not made us happier. I am firmly convinced that when we learn how to listen to people and to their stories, we will be able to hear the real needs and the real wants. Most people are reasonable and concerned for others as much as for themselves. If they are not, then by listening to them we may actually give them the best tool to learn this for themselves. If we go on as we are now, then healthcare will literally ruin the industrialised nations with its demands for ever more money spent on ever more and often useless tests and treatments. We cannot afford not to listen. Only when we listen do we hear what a person needs, that is, what holistic care may involve.

Listening takes time and it takes people. It takes human contact and willingness, and need to be human with each other more than patients and professionals, clients and therapists, or whatever other divisions there are between people. We need to hear what our children are saying because they have a lot of simple wisdom which we tend to dismiss as immature but may be more a reflection of our own insecurity. We need above all to hear what older people are saying. With the increasing number of older people we need to re-think radically how we treat older people. At present, we have the rather schizophrenic situation where we can prolong life considerably, but we do not at the same time value the life we prolong. Ethics, morality, and health care are not necessarily walking in step. That may not always be a bad thing as all ethics is formed at the edge of the possible. What we need to do, though, is dare to be courageous with the kind of care we can, want and need to give.

I have yet another postcard of an impossible image. This time it is a man riding a monocycle on a telegraph wire on a foggy day with a very pale sun high in the sky. The man seems to enjoy himself. Holistic care is something like this picture: it is daring, unrealistic, unknown and unclear, even mad when looked at rationally. It is only in the doing of it that it becomes possible. Each time we achieve something like holistic care, however, we know that we have advanced humanity, and that, after all, is what it is really about.

I doubt if our systems of healthcare will or even can switch to a truly holistic way of working, but it must surely be the ideal. You will have gathered that I have not been able to describe or define holistic care. At the end of this paper, the best that I can say is that holistic care is what the patient or client needs it to be. It is what emerges when professionals and clients talk, listen, and share their needs, possibilities, and gift. When both client and practitioner are enriched and both feel 'healed', although only one of them may have been looking for it, we as practitioners will indeed have been acting ethically and holistically.

CHAPTER FOUR

Ethical Considerations in the Allocation of Resources in Healthcare

Marianne Arndt

Introduction

Approaching the biotech century, as the twenty-first century has been described, it may well be worthwhile examining the meaning of such a term in the context of resource allocation in healthcare.

Limited resources in healthcare and their just distribution are topics of immanent public concern. Money, time, energy, and space need to be managed wisely and allocated justly, where disease and suffering are concerned. This is not just a question of economic or moral principles and their application to healthcare settings. In my paper, I focus on the specific plea of nurses and of nursing over the meaning of what it costs to care for people who are unwell.

After defining the terms justice, equality and healthcare resources, I give a general overview of the contemporary discussion. Several questions seem to be of concern in the area of healthcare economics:

How much money is to be spent on healthcare?

How is this money to be allocated within the health services?

What is available for use by healthcare providers? (What is it that money can buy?)

How are decisions to be made?

Answers to the first and second questions have political implications and lead to general deliberations about social justice. Answers are influenced by priorities, which a people will set. Such priorities depend on the perceived meanings of cultural, historical, social and personal aspects. But in the face of an overwhelming availability of technological options in the medical arena, it may no longer be a question of how much money is to be spent, but rather: Can we pay for what we can do? The third question defines the options actually available, it relates to:

Medical technology in the fields of diagnostics and therapy,
Pharmacological options,
Buildings and other spaces,
People managing the first three items above,
People and their physical presence,
Information technology.

Information technology is needed to utilise all aspects mentioned and it may be noted that this has climbed to the top of most budgets.

The last question, 'How are decisions to be made?' is the main concern of this paper. I suggest that three main perspectives will help us to provide answers to some of the problems in the area of healthcare resource allocation. Firstly, the understanding that decisions cannot fruitfully be made hypothetically by so called specialists; we need the public debate. Secondly, the value perception of health will have to include a spiritual element; a purely materialistic basis for the process of decision-making cannot serve a people. Thirdly, value perceptions are subject to practical learning, the implementation of which could be crucial to the aforementioned public debate.

I regard nursing as an inherently moral activity. Thus, I am concerned with the money, time, energy, and space that nurses have at their disposal within the overall allocation of healthcare resources. I argue a case for greater emphasis to be placed on human resources in our heathcare systems in Europe as opposed to the seemingly unlimited development of medical technology.

Some Propositions

It seems that the term healthcare is quite inappropriate for the realities of our present-day healthcare systems. Health may be the focus of such systems but care, defined as caring for and being with people, most certainly is not the main item on the political agendas of most countries when looked at from the expenditure point of view. Furthermore, even though the focus of our health systems may appear to be the wellbeing of people, I want to ask cautiously if it is not that the human need of people is being exploited by the implicitly conveyed objective of health, ability, activity and productivity?

The technological options of medical treatments that are on offer seem to have turned into an end in themselves. They no longer appear to be the means to the end of better health. The background for this shift may be found in the power of the international medical technological and pharmacological industries as well as in the competitive structures of the medical academic establishment.

I quote the remarks of a young aspiring medical professor, which was made two years ago during the faculty board meeting at one of the medical faculties in Berlin, Germany. He said, 'Do we want to degenerate into an Infirmary looking after the chronically sick? Do we want to give up our scientific ambitions? We have got to hold on to what we have achieved so far, no other considerations must interfere with our research objectives'.

These words were said during a debate about the proposed closing of a heart transplantation centre. The centre had been initiated and financed for a university hospital in the former East Berlin three years previously. To give you the whole story: immediately after unification, some health centres in East Berlin had been closed and others were being invested in order to equalise services and to concentrate resources. In the course of restructuring the health services in Berlin, one of the health centres was transformed into a special care cardiac unit with heart transplantation facilities. In spite of a well established transplantation centre in a West Berlin university clinic and in spite of the recently opened cardiac unit in the East, the first mentioned university had managed to procure the resources for the third centre now to be closed by the Senate. 'Do we want to degenerate into an Infirmary?' This was clear and open speak, and it was applauded by the generally rather disinterested members of the faculty board. This is just one instance of how priorities are set. There are many more examples, and not only in Germany.

In a way, it may be said that together with the implicit promise of wellbeing and of health, we are supplied with goods we cannot really afford. Of course, medical technology and pharmacology have brought about blessings for humankind, which we could never have dreamt of. Medicine may be seen as a blessing for the development of our civilisations. The same achievements, however, which allow more people to overcome formerly fatal illnesses or injuries are the cause of an ever increasing ageing population. To reach the age of a hundred is becoming increasingly common. But we also have increasingly chronically ill elderly people whose care causes a strain on the healthcare services. Thus, the blessings of biotechnology in combination with other factors such as better nutritional options, vaccinations, and a generally improved standard of living, confront us with new problems.

Fewer people with productive capacities will have to pay for the goods of welfare states for more people who are not in the work process any more. Obviously, health can no longer be seen as the means by which we secure productivity.

At various levels, we sense the spectre of gross injustice in the distribution of healthcare resources. What concerns me as a nurse, is that the element of care may be lost from our health services. I hold, firstly, that health must be attainable by all, irrespective of status, age, race, etc. With this, I repeat a statement of the *WHO Constitution*. I hold, secondly, that health is not only dependent on medical technology and, thirdly, that health has a spiritual dimension. From this, it follows that a new awareness for the human encounter can help us to overcome some of the problems which arise for a just distribution of healthcare resources. This, I will argue and unfold in the course of this paper.

Definitions

I use the word 'justice' in the platonic sense of the cardinal virtue. It is a prerequisite for all human interactions. This applies to legal justice as much as it does to distributive justice. Here, of course, we are only concerned with the latter in the sense of social justice. I also understand justice as fairness, as Rawls decrees, allowing each member of a given society the same liberty as any other. As an ensuing consequence, applying a principle of equity, the access to the available goods of society must be granted to all its members.

When talking about healthcare resources I am not thinking of the technological and pharmacological goods only. When looking at medico-technological means in the hands of healthcare professionals, these professionals need to be in the centre of the picture. In the current bioethical debate, both aspects, that of justice and that of healthcare resources, are discussed controversially. For the last twelve years, this debate has been on the agenda of politicians, philosophers and medical professionals. The public is now slowly taking it up. And in the public arena, such debate finds its most appropriate place, as we shall see in the course of my presentation.

To quote from a current seminal text in the area of healthcare ethics: 'Society must be consulted and debate the criteria upon which resource allocations are to be made' (Singleton, J. and McLaren, S., *Ethical Foundations of Healthcare*, p. 133). Singleton and McLaren also demand that: 'Above all, healthcare practitioners, economists, and managers must be educated to reason morally. This is a vital prerequisite for the delivery of high quality health-care in a just society' (Singleton, J. and McLaren, S., *Ethical Foundations of Healthcare*, p. 133).

It may be one of the most important misconceptions about the meaning of professional expertise that it is enough to know how. We cannot neglect the moral knowledge that is needed for making moral decisions. Perhaps it was because of a lack in this latter field that it was possible for the so-called medical model to take precedence in our health services and the care element to be so neglected. Perhaps it was this lack which caused the German doctors to fight for their third heart transplantation centre in Berlin.

Controversial Discussions

1. Consequentialist approaches:

The main controversy in the healthcare resource allocation debate is that between a utilitarian approach and a deontological stance. The health economist Alan Williams proposed a rational approach, which is supposed to give a just measurement for the allocation of resources. The system is based on a utilitarian principle of cost-effectiveness. Effectivity is measured by the quality of life years to be expected as a result of any medical intervention. The criteria for the measurement of quality are determined by the expected degree of freedom from pain and disability. Worked into the calculation are the expected numbers of years a patient will live after a given intervention (Williams, 'Economics, Society and Healthcare Ethics' in *Principles of Healthcare Ethics*). Thus, Williams, describing the concept of Quality Adjusted Life Years (QALY), says: 'The general idea is that a beneficial healthcare activity is one that generates a positive amount of Qaly's, and that an efficient healthcare activity is one where the cost per Qaly is as low as it can be' (Seedhouse, D., *Ethics – The Heart of Healthcare*, p. 120).

For example:

Heart transplantation valued at 4.5, Qaly's costing £ 5,000

Kidney transplantation valued at 5, Qaly's costing £ 3,000

A hip replacement valued at 4, Qaly's costing £ 750

Williams says further: 'A high priority healthcare activity is one where the cost per Qaly is low, and a low priority activity is one where the cost per Qaly is high.' (Seedhouse, D., *Ethics – The Heart of Healthcare*, p. 120) The hip transplantation would be the most efficient activity and have high priority.

Can we adjust our priorities only according to cost and according to the easily measurable values of freedom from pain and mobility? The evaluation of presence or absence of both may differ enormously among individuals and further they cannot be the only arbiters in any judgement about life quality. A 55 year old woman, living with multiple sclerosis, will see and understand disability and ability in quite a different light than an active member of an octogenarian running club.

Still, the consequence of such calculation demonstrates a sense for justice if seen in the light of macroallocation. In summer 1995, we heard that the new South African Government decreed the suspension of expensive transplantation surgery. Organ transplantation can obviously not improve the overall health status of a given population, as they are needed only for a select few. As to the South African situation, a comparative figure was given to justify the decision. This reads that the cost of one heart transplantation equals roughly the cost of antibiotic treatment for possibly fatal pneumonia in 25,000 small children (Arndt, *Ethik denken – Maßstäbe zum Handeln in der Pflege*, p. 127).

A cost-benefit calculation may provide a number of advantages, which seem to point to an overall system of justice. But *in extremis*, quoting Veatch, it can be hypothesised that the greatest benefit – that is the greatest amount of happiness – would be achieved if one per cent of the population were excluded from healthcare and this one per cent were to be made up by the extremely ill, and by the chronically ill, both groups using up the greatest part of available resources (Veatch, *A Theory of Medical Ethics*, p. 172).

2. *Deontological approaches:*
The healthcare resource debate is, however, looking at alternatives from utilitarian approaches. One such alternative was seen in randomisation. (Harris, *The Value of Life*) In situations where either-or decisions appear inevitable lots could be drawn. Such an approach seems to hold that the present technology-oriented stance in medicine must need be lived to the full. That is, what is possible must be on offer, and if the blanket is too short, either feet or head will have to freeze.

On quite different lines, value priorities as decisive moments could be arrived at by the involvement of the public. This was practised with the so-called Oregon plan. In 1993, the Federal Government of the State of Oregon passed a programme that intended to make adequate healthcare available to all citizens of the State including those below the federal poverty line. This made the rationing of provisions necessary. Involving a process of public debate, decisions were made as to which treatments or procedures should be available (Minogue, *Bioethics – A Committee Approach*, p. 250). Thus value priorities were being stated. Public opinion favoured preventative healthcare programmes and antenatal support over high-technology treatments or expensive support of premature babies with poor survival chances (Singleton, J. and McLaren, S., *Ethical Foundations of Healthcare*, p. 132).

In Switzerland, a serious debate has started on the rationing of medical treatments. A manifesto for fair distribution of means in the health services has been published. It contains recommendations to increase the personal contribution for preventive therapeutics and demands that new therapeutic methods should be introduced more reluctantly but that the testing of the effectiveness of standard treatments should have research priorities (Köchli, D.I., *Ein Heisses Eisen*). A democratic debate is called for. The public will have to be involved in the development of criteria for the distribution of healthcare resources.

In 1989, Lewis and Cherney conducted an opinion survey in selected North American States. It appeared that the majority of the sample would select younger in preference to older persons in order to benefit from expensive health treatments. This would suggest that society operates a utilitarian approach to access scarce medical resources (Singleton, J. and McLaren, S., *Ethical Foundations of Healthcare*, p. 132). In understanding justice as fairness we may be confronted with the problem of prevalent societal values which may not be in favour of the older, the weaker, the poorer, and the less intelligent. One of the authors of the Swiss manifesto stated that solidarity with the vulnerable members of society must never be sacrificed. Still, the distribution of healthcare resources does appear to be a societal question. It is neither a burden for professionals nor their privilege to make decisions in this area. The expression of prevalent societal values must be given a chance to come to the fore. Maybe societal values will have to change? Possibly, this is a major area for the activities of health educators, healthcare workers, ethicists, and politicians.

A Personalised View
So far, I have looked at the question of resource allocation from a rather impersonal stance. Ethical decisions in the areas of healthcare will always involve real people. Real people have to make specific decisions in actual situations. We may debate the problems concerned with the allocation of resources from a general institutional or political perspective, but it is in the personal encounter at the microlevel that the lack of resources is sorely felt by patients and is coped with by staff.

There is Mrs Libby, a 55-year-old lady. Over five years ago, multiple sclerosis was diagnosed. During a remission in her condition, she had spent a good summer at home being looked after by her husband, her sister and the community nurse. A routine examination had revealed cervical cancer and she has now been admitted to hospital for a hysterectomy. Mrs Libby, Monica, has had good support from her whole family during the difficult time of diagnosis and decision-making. Charge Nurse O'Connor, Joan, is giving out evening medications on the gynaecological ward. She enters Monica's sideroom and finds her crying. This was nothing really unusual considering the situation. But Nurse O'Connor has the medicines to finish, has to prepare three further ladies for theatre in the morning, has to get the handover for the nightshift ready, as well as all the paperwork for tomorrow's operation list (Monica is among the patients due for theatre), and an emergency patient with a spontaneous abortion has just been admitted and Charge Nurse should also do a reflective session with the student nurse before going off duty.

I do not have to describe the work pressures of a busy gynaecological ward in more detail. But here is Monica, sitting in a chair beside her bed with tears running down her face. Nurse O'Connor stands in the door, the student behind her peeping into the room. Once again, this nurse, Joan, feels her inability to do what she knows would be right at this moment. But there simply is no time to sit down with Monica, to listen to her slurred, slow speech, to hold her hand, to be with her. Instead she can only give her a compassionate look, hand her the pills and say, 'I'll be back before I go off, student is going to help you with these pills.'

It is such scenarios that make us feel the cruelty of our health-care systems. (The nurse could actually be Johanna, or Jean, or José there is not much difference as to staff shortage in Europe.) Our systems are geared towards throughput, towards the effective use of time, space, personnel, and equipment. The beds are allocated, use must be made of diagnostic technology, and operating theatres must never be empty. The running of a hospital is a logistic masterpiece and the people involved have to succumb to the regimen of financial priorities.

A new nuclear spin tomography unit has been installed in a given hospital, a large sum of money been spent, but the calculations did not include extra staff to comfort those who through the benefit of diagnostic competence are confronted with personal catastrophe. No extra time, no extra staff is allocated to be with people like Monica.

Health and Values

The basis of healthcare has two elements. One is a medico-technical and the other a relational one. Both elements are dependent upon each other. In the question of resource allocation, it is not enough to discuss the material perspective regarding the availability of technological means or of pharmaceutical options. The nurse taking medication to a patient may well make the difference between its effectiveness and its uselessness. Thinking of Monica and Joan O'Connor, this becomes obvious.

Care is not only the administration of therapeutic means.

Care is relationship and as such, it has in itself therapeutic value. No health system can claim the care attribute if the central meaning of the human encounter is not recognised. This encounter happens at a personal level and it is greatly independent of medical technology and of pharmacology, providing human resources are basically available. The involvement of people in the healthcare services includes nurses, other health workers, hospital chaplains, but also volunteers, family and friends.

Communication and Ethics

Communication appeared as a buzzword in the late 60s and in the 70s. The cry for better and more effective communication resulted in the training and preparation of professional communicators. No doubt, the importance of effective communication cannot be underestimated, but communication as such has so far not solved societal problems. We may, however, be more aware of our problems because of more effective communication media.

Ethics was the new buzzword of the 80s and 90s in the UK and in Europe. Moral philosophy was seemingly discovered then. A perceived lack of ethical content was compensated by a prolific output in ethics books and articles. In all areas of healthcare, ethics was emphasised and included in curricula. Universities started to offer degree courses in healthcare ethics and indeed an ever-growing body of experts entered an increasingly more complex bioethics debate. Again, our problems became more obvious, but they were not solved because more experts knew more about ethics. Both communication and ethics seemed no more than fashionable areas of interest. But communication for its own sake is empty, and an ethics which does not include action must be futile.

It is indeed not enough to seek solutions to our problems by employing varied techniques of either communication or of philosophical deliberation. We need a value system that will allow us to shift the focus of attention from more and increasingly sophisticated technology as an end in itself to the personal. The

WHO endorsed its Constitution from 1948 where the General Assembly stated that it is one of the fundamental rights of every human being to attain the enjoyment of the highest standard of health (World Health Organisation, *Constitution*, 1948).

In a paper given at a symposium on medical ethics last year in Davos, Derek Yach, a WHO official, said that 'health for all remains an enduring vision ... recognising the oneness of humanity and therefore the need to promote health and to alleviate ill health and suffering universally and in the spirit of solidarity ... The vision is based on the following key values:

1. Recognition of the highest attainable standard of health as a fundamental right;

2. Continued and strengthened application of ethics to health policy, research and service provision;

3. Implementation of equity-oriented policies;

4. Incorporation of a gender perspective into health policies and strategies' (Yach, *Ethik in Der Medizin*, 10 (Supplement) p. 11).

Yach invoked the Golden Rule and called for collective action. For far too long medical ethics has been concerned with principles as its basis. John Finnis, Professor of Law and Legal Philosophy at Oxford claims: 'The principles ... are matters for moral philosophy. But reason's full implications, and morality's practical applications, are well understood only when full account is taken of the human situation' (Finnis, J. and Fisher, A., 'The Four Principles and Their Use' in *Principles of Healthcare Ethics*, p. 31). Finnis refers to the Georgetown Mantra, the rights oriented principles of autonomy, beneficence, non-maleficence, and justice.

The philosopher Jürgen Habermas, influenced by the feminist critic Seyla Benhabib (Horster, *Habermas zur Einführung*), expounded an ethics concerned with communicative action. Here, different sets of guidelines come to the fore. Habermas advocates an ethics of discourse, the elements of which would be:

1. Solidarity as empathy and compassion;

2. Co-operation instead of autonomy (which stands in danger to leave a patient entirely to his own (impaired) resources);

3. Community with those we care for;

4. Communication which is also prepared to be silent.

In order to preserve the caring element in our health system, emphasis needs to shift from technological resources as ends to resources as means. Technology is permeating our lives and our world, but the human encounter cannot ever be replaced by technology. It can be enhanced, however, if we use our resources – that is ourselves – wisely. Joan, Johanna, Jean, or José, the nurses in our story, want to be with Monica in order to give value to the use of medical technology, in order to provide a communicative basis for the medication that Monica is getting.

The human situation is of importance and not an abstract application of principles. It is the personal human encounter which needs to be considered too when deliberating about our caring resources. It is in the context of the life-world of sickness, of frailty, and of suffering that decisions have to originate. Thus, the compassionate being with a patient can be teaching us priorities; a co-operative spirit amongst all healthcare workers should further mutual understanding against a competitive staking out of claims for the furtherance of a professional profile; the perusal of communitarian structures where all members of a given society have equal opportunity and freedom to be heard could help us on the road to just distribution of healthcare resources; and finally the communicative exchange about the moral requirements of our age and time could assure the prerequisite for wise decision-making in this difficult field.

A Nursing Perspective

As I am a nurse, and as nurses are those people in the health services that spend the most time with patients, I will for the remaining part of this paper concentrate my emphasis on the situation of nurses.

The nurse-patient encounter is embedded within an institutional framework. This framework functions according to the dictating rules of commercialism. The demand of the medical establishment is, for most nurses in Europe, still the decisive impetus for action. (Monica would not be in hospital if there was no operation pending, and it is the physician who looks after the MS side of her medical needs and prescribes her tablets.) A nurse will get a great deal of her recognition by the competent handling of medico-technical apparatuses and pharmaceutical applications. Thus, nurse education until recently had been driven exclusively by a natural science approach. The medical model fashioned nursing curricula and, indeed, in many European countries this is still the case. Although 'nursing science' has made its appearance, and contents taken from the social sciences enrich nursing education, the medical model seems imprinted in the minds of many nurses, nurse teachers, and of young student nurses too.

However, a start has been made. In the United Kingdom nursing is developing into a discipline of its own right, which should be studied in pre-registration university courses. Scotland has adopted a policy where nurse education is being transferred into the academic realm. In Ireland, a change is proposed which looks at nursing as an all graduate profession. The Report of the Commission on Nursing advocates pre-registration nursing education at degree-level in institutions of tertiary education (Government of the Republic of Ireland, *Report of The Commission on Nursing,* (Rep. Com.), p. 79). It is recommended that the future framework for the pre-registration education of nurses be based on a four-year degree programme. Such a step shows the recognition of the need for more than a 'trained nurse' who can carry out medical orders. The Report states: 'The rationale for integrating pre-registration nursing education into the third-level sector at degree level was identified as the need to prepare nurses better for an ever more complex and technological system of health provision.'

Here, it is clearly recognised that the advancement of technology has changed the requirement in nurse education. It is hoped that the allusion to an ever more complex system of health provision includes the deeper understanding of the complexity of human relationships.

The consultative process, which led to the Report, has revealed a need for the greater involvement of nurses and midwives in planning and policy development. This statement clearly indicates an appreciation of the role of nurses and of midwives within the totality of the health provision services. The voices of nurses and of midwives need to be heard where healthcare is concerned. More and better technology does not simply mean the need to secure more financial means to obtain and to maintain such technology. It also means the need for more human resources. More well educated nurses and midwives are needed in order to mediate between suffering individuals and the employed technology. Healthcare workers' dissatisfaction is often routed in this area of want. The demands of technology or of medical routine take over and Nurse O'Connor will have to leave a student with Monica. No time is left for the human encounter.

The involvement of nurses and midwives in policy-making and especially in the participation in the overall financial planning of the health services provided is said to be of greatest importance in the Report. The Report says also that matrons '... should be given more explicit input into the determination of the budget and greater control and responsibility over its utilisation (Government of the Republic of Ireland, *Report of The Commission on Nursing*, (Rep. Com.), p. 129). Such nursing input, it would be hoped, should counterbalance the technological overburden and bring further human resources to bear upon the caring aspects of a health system. A further sentence in this context gives rise to great hopes: The Commission recommends that the Department of Health and Children, health service providers and nursing organisations examine the development of appropriate systems to determine staffing levels (Government of the Republic of Ireland, *Report of The Commission on Nursing*, (Rep. Com.), p. 138). The Report of the Commission indicates that a consultative process is in motion. Such a process – if it is to be effective – is to be initiated at the highest political level (as the Commission Report was). Here lies the ethical responsibility of government, but it has to be expanded and reach every healthcare practitioner as well.

Caring as a Societal Value
Thus far, we have seen that the responsibility for a just distribution of resources is divided and lies at different levels. We have examined an example of governmental involvement of recent import in this country. We have also seen that priorities can be set at the institutional levels of decision-making; and I have demonstrated that it is at the personal level in the direct encounter that resource allocation comes to bear.

In examining some models of decision-making in the area of resource allocation, I have pointed out the need for public involvement. I have drawn attention to the arbitrariness of public opinion. But I wish to make a further point as to possible perspectives for the future of healthcare. Geoff Hunt, in a recent paper, wrote the most enlightening sentence: 'A purely rational (philosophical, bioethical) foundation for the rightness or wrongness of abortion (or anything else) is impossible. If science, particularly sociology and psychology, had not given religious and moral attitudes such a bad press, we might be looking in the right direction for such foundation' (Hunt, G., 'Abortion: Why Bioethics Have No Answer', *Nursing Ethics*, p. 57).

During the latest WHO General Assembly in May last year a new emphasis was put upon the fact that a valid and workable definition of health must include reference to spiritual aspects of health and to moral values. Thus, the General Assembly in developing a new global health policy acknowledges the uniqueness of each person and the need to respond to each individual's quest for meaning, purpose and belonging.

When thinking in terms of spiritual values, it may well be worthwhile addressing the fact that as human beings we are finite and live in a finite world. We will have to accept that our resources in all areas are finite too. Possibly, it is of value to consider the meaning of fasting in the light of the distribution of healthcare resources. Possibly fasting could have a societal dimension in the context of our topic – that is: abstinence from some therapeutic goods. Spirituality begins, however, at the interpersonal level in the intimate communicative exchange. Such exchange would have to start in the private sphere of spiritual counselling but could involve healthcare workers, as well as hospital chaplains, parish priests, and pastors. Considering a new approach to fasting could be relevant to expenditure within our healthcare services, and should then be part of a public debate. This societal dimension will have to include the fact that there is gross injustice in our world at a global level concerning the distribution of goods.

Health is seen as a great value, but its meaning is really understood only when we experience its lack. At most times we are not aware of our precariousness and of our human vulnerability. We are, however, exposed to suffering because of injury, illness, and death. We will have to submit to the feebleness of our existence and will have to include it in the picture of our reality.

Some of us have had to do this early. Others have been shaped later in life by devastating experiences of disease and death. But most of us have also experienced the healing presence and the comforting power of human caring, be it in the voluntary sector or in the organised healthcare services. Basically most of us are aware of the importance of such services. I have spoken about the need for solidarity and I have mentioned that the main problem is not that our resources in the healthcare services are scarce, but that our allocation criteria and priorities are not adequate. To quote Seedhouse: '… since 'scarce resources' are scarce only as a result of lack of funds that might be available from other sources, and since by the use of statistics it is possible to predict fairly accurately how many dialysis machines and other such resources will be needed, it should become public knowledge that lives are being lost and those doctors who must decide are being placed in impossible positions as a result of human priorities, not natural circumstances' (Seedhouse, D., *Ethics – The Heart of Healthcare*, p. 126).

We live in this world and not in any other. In healthcare, we deal with human beings and not any other beings. If we want just healthcare allocation systems, we will have to produce them ourselves. Compassion, community, co-operation, and communication cannot simply be demanded and will not just appear, because Habermas, Benhabib, and some other moral philosophers thought and wrote about their importance. They will have to be learned. In the Aristotelian sense of practical wisdom or *phronesis*, I am not leading a good life because I know something about the values that can determine a good life. It is the practice which is needed. Aristotle located the source of ethical insight in experience itself. Knowing how to act, the possession of practical wisdom, means having an eye for solutions; and that can only be developed through a combination of training in the right habits and direct acquaintance with practical situations (Rowe, C., 'Ethics in Ancient Greece' in *A Companion to Ethics*).

In our context, I would propose (in addition to sending nursing students to university) that it might do something toward changing societal values to bring nursing as a subject into primary schools, secondary and high schools. Nursing or practical caring should be taught and experienced, enhancing and developing already present aptitudes which take heed of human vulnerability and of suffering. Momentarily children are confronted with the basic elements of economics, technology, and commercialism. The values of interest for later life are being inculcated as early as Kindergarten age. Why should not the values of solidarity, of compassion, and care, and an early understanding for human vulnerability supply and complete the preparation for adult responsibilities?

Not that everyone needs to be a nurse or a medical doctor. The economist, the bank manager, and the journalist are important people influencing public opinion. And if it does come to the democratic process, the discursive public debate, practical wisdom as to health and as to care cannot be amiss. If the resource allocation discussion is to include the public, a public value system that includes a sense of solidarity and an intimate understanding of suffering could assure decisions which make for justice and for peace.

Conclusion

In the approaching biotech century, it is of immanent importance to convey an understanding of the human condition as vulnerable and precarious. Technology cannot work without human mediation. Healthcare workers have to be aware of their human role as mediators. Nurses may have to learn anew that human presence has therapeutic value, but it is also the structures of healthcare services that need to be looked at anew. Institutional structures can be basically just or unjust, morally good or bad. Still, it is not enough to see the probelms of just distribution of resources from personal or local institutional and local political perspectives. A global view will have to guide political decisions. We may have to re-think the structures of our institutions and include the pleas of poorer countries in our deliberations about just distributions of healthcare resources.

We will not attain social justice if technological progress is understood as the main source for health, and if medico-technological means are on offer for a lucky few only. We will have to re-evaluate the meaning of human dignity. This includes the personal encounter and a spiritual dimension. Do we want health at all cost? Becoming more aware of the deep value of the direct human touch, we may wish to invest more in the abilities of people to be with people. And that may be more affordable for all.

CHAPTER FIVE

Autonomy and Consent

Denis A. Cusack

Any discussion of autonomy and consent in healthcare decisions must give due consideration to the medical, ethical and legal aspects of the healthcare provider-patient relationship. It is a relationship that is inherently unequal, but not withstanding that inequality, there are well recognised legal and ethical rights and duties of both parties to the relationship. The manner in which society assesses the value of human life is fundamental to this consideration. Does society attribute an absolute intrinsic value to each human life regardless of the means or cost of preserving or prolonging that life? Or does society adopt a utilitarian approach and assess value of a life based on its subjective or objective value?

The concept of patient autonomy is now frequently referred to. There is a much greater focus on the patient as a person and on the legal and ethical basis for the healthcare provider-patient relationship. Nowhere is this concept of patient autonomy tested as rigorously as in the area of consent to medical intervention and, increasingly, patient refusal. There must be recognition of both rights and duties on the part of patient and healthcare provider. The very concept of autonomy is not one for which there is a uniform definition. It has been variously defined as the right to self-govern, or the right to partial self-government, or the right to self-determination.

The moral basis of the healthcare provider-patient relationship through the centuries has been the Hippocratic Oath and its successor declarations of Geneva, Helsinki, and Tokyo. Healthcare professions also have professional codes set out by the relevant statutory or voluntary regulators of those professions, as for example *A Guide to Ethical Conduct and Behaviour* issued by the Medical Council of Ireland for registered medical practitioners. These various codes must inform and be coupled with the individual healthcare provider's conscience.

The legal basis for the relationship is a combination of international laws, fundamental rights, the law of tort and the law of contract. The patient is usually in a triangular legal relationship within the health services involving the institution, the healthcare provider, and patient. In a wholly private arrangement between healthcare provider and patient, the law of contract will be of relevance. However, courts would usually have greater regard to the law of tort, or wrongdoing, in a dispute between healthcare provider and patient where there is an allegation relating to the proper standard of care provided. Nonetheless, in the real world, the basis for this relationship must recognise an inherent and perhaps insurmountable inequality between the parties. Healthcare providers and senior doctors, in particular, have status, knowledge, and experience in their specialist fields and may appear quite formidable to the patient. The patient is vulnerable, dependent and in relative ignorance. These characteristics are not unique to the healthcare provider-patient relationship. They are characteristic of many professional-client relationships. The protection of the vulnerable person generally is contained in that branch of law pertaining to fiduciary relationships that arises from the idea of trust. In the Court of Appeals, State of Washington, it was stated (Miller v Kennedy):

> 'the duty of the doctor to inform the patient is a fiduciary duty. The patient is entitled to rely upon the physician to tell him what he needs to know about the condition of his own body. The patient has a right to chart his own destiny, and the doctor must supply the patient with the material facts the patient will need in order to intelligently chart that destiny with dignity.'

When it comes to issues as fundamental as health or life, the patient is especially, and anxiously, vulnerable.

The legalistic concept of consent can be explained quite readily by using the term 'agreement'. This recognises that there must be an opportunity given to the patient to agree to medical intervention and also a right to disagree. In order for there to be a legally valid consent, the patient must have legal capacity, must give consent voluntarily, and must be informed. Legal capacity is intrinsic to any consideration of the concept of autonomy and is assessed by reference to the status of the patient by age or mental capacity. An adult is presumed to have such capacity and the Non-Fatal Offences Against the Person Act 1997 recognises a minor of 16 years or older in the same manner. A second method of assessing capacity is by reference to the ability of the person to understand the consent process rather than by strict reference to status only. Increasingly, the courts are applying a combination of the two tests. The Canadian case of Reibl v Hughes (1980) stated simply that law on capacity focuses on 'the patient's ability to understand the information given and to decide rationally.'

The UK Law Commission's recommendations on consent include a proposal which essentially codifies a ruling of the Law Lords in the Gillick case:

'a person should be regarded as being unable to make a decision by reason of age or immaturity if at the time a decision needs to be made, he/she does not have sufficient understanding and intelligence to understand the information relevant to the decision, including information about the reasonably foreseeable consequences of deciding one way or another or of failing to make that decision.'

The legal right of the patient to refuse is based on Article 40.3.1 of Bunreacht na hÉireann, provided that the legal criteria of capacity, voluntariness, and being informed are fulfilled. In circumstances where a patient refuses life-saving treatment that is not considered burdensome by others, and the courts are asked to consider the refusal, great attention will be paid to these three criteria. There are of course occasions when non-consensual treatment may be permitted as in an emergency when the patient is unconscious or incompetent under certain provisions of the mental health and public health laws and where there is a real and imminent danger to another person. The situation becomes more complex if a second life is directly involved, as in pregnancy, and courts throughout the world have had to balance the rights of a woman to have her wish for non-intervention respected with those of the child *in utero* to receive life-saving treatment through the mother.

However, the paternalistic approach to informed consent can no longer be acceptable in Irish medical law. The most extreme form of paternalism is the imposition of treatment or intervention by the doctor against the patient's objection. In its most benign form, it is the application of orthodox negligence principles whereby reference is made to the general and approved practice of what a doctor would usually tell a patient. In the extreme application of the 'prudent patient test', a patient would be informed of every conceivable eventuality. That extreme is as unacceptable as the extreme paternalistic approach. In the Canadian case of McInerney v MacDonald, the Supreme Court held that flowing from the patient-doctor relationship there was a duty on the doctor to make 'proper disclosure' to the patient.

If a patient is to be 'informed', then he or she must be capable of understanding his medical condition at a basic level and of comprehending the nature, scope, and significance of any proposed intervention. The doctor must explain the aims of the treatment, any discomfort, side effects, or risks that might be reasonably foreseeable. Any alternatives or choices of intervention must be explained and the patient must be free to refuse or withdraw from treatment at any reasonable time. One of the problems of informed consent arises when there is a mismatch of expectations between the healthcare provider and the patient. There has been a move from applying the 'reasonable doctor' test only to the application of this test combined with a 'reasonable patient' approach. Thus general and approved professional practice must be considered in combination with the rights of a patient.

Where there is a medical necessity for therapeutic intervention, it is general and approved practice not to disclose minimal risks which might cause unnecessary anxiety and stress to the patient and might deter the patient from undergoing the necessary treatment. When the nature of the procedure is such that it is not a medical necessity but an elective intervention, as with many cases of sterilisation and cosmetic surgery, different considerations arise. In Walsh v Family Planning Clinic (1992), which involved elective vasectomy, it was stated 'that the risk ... however exceptional or remote ... of grave consequences ... should be explained in the clearest language'. Material risks would include those which are minor but frequent or which are major but infrequent. In the American case of Canterbury v Spence (1972) it was properly stated that 'there is no bright line separating the significant from the insignificant; the answer in each case must abide rule of reason'. Indeed, the prudent patient approach in Canterbury recognised the legitimacy of non-disclosure on grounds of necessity or therapeutic privilege.

In Rogers v Whitaker (1992), an Australian case, it was stated that the provision of information is part of 'a single comprehensive duty covering all the ways in which a doctor is to exercise his skill and judgement'. It further stated:

'the law should recognise that a doctor has a duty to warn a patient of a material risk inherent in the proposed treatment; a risk is material if, in the circumstances of the particular case, a reasonable person in the patient's position, if warned of the risk would be likely to attach significance to it, or if the medical practitioner is or should reasonably be likely to attach significance to it, or if the medical practitioner is or should reasonably be aware that the particular patient, if warned of the risk, would be likely to attach significance to it.'

The imparting of information must always be in a sensitive and caring manner as part of professional healthcare rather than merely a legalistic fulfilling of legal duties.

A Guide to Ethical Conduct and Behaviour from the Medical Council of Ireland (1998) states that it would 'be reasonable to assume … tacit consent'. The legal basis for this assertion is dubious and it would have been more proper to refer to implied rather than tacit consent. The Guidelines recognise the right to refuse consent and set out the caution required in particular circumstances such as the unconscious patient, the violent patient, the mentally ill, the mentally handicapped and children. Consent given on behalf of a child by a parent or a person *in loco parentis* or on behalf of a ward of court is well recognised in law. Consent given by a spouse or next-of-kin on behalf of a person incapable of consenting due to unconsciousness is also recognised in law but it is not without difficulties in all cases. The law in relation to consent on behalf of an adult who is not a ward of court or who is not in an emergency situation requires clarification.

The advance directive, also known as the living will or anticipatory decision, brings the whole question of patient autonomy into even starker consideration. Its status in law is that it would be recognised provided it fulfilled the criteria for validity: that the person was competent, informed and was under no undue influence and that the directive was current and specific to the circumstances in which the patient is. Although there are no statutory provisions, if those criteria were fulfilled, then there is little doubt that there would be a valid advance directive, assuming of course that the instructions contained therein were not unlawful. However, the question of enforceability of such directive where it was contrary to the ethical principles of an institution or individual healthcare provider is a matter of serious doubt.

Where the patient is not competent to make such a decision this is where the most acute questions as to patient autonomy arise. Combinations of the best interest test and a substituted judgement test are often used in this circumstance. The former is very much a test based on the paternalistic approach whereby other people make decisions based on what they believe to be in the patient's best interest. The latter test is one in which somebody puts themselves in the shoes of the patient, so to speak, and attempts to arrive at a decision that it is believed the patient would make if competent.

It is in the case where self-determination or the decision of others come into conflict with medical opinions and decisions that the Courts have intervened. In *Re T* (1992), perhaps the clearest statement of patient autonomy was given:

'the patient's interest consists of his right to self-determination – his right to live his own life as he wishes even it would damage his health or lead to his premature death. Society's interest is in upholding the concept that all human life is sacred and that it should be preserved if at all possible. It is well established that in the ultimate the right of the individual is paramount.'

It was also stated in that case that

'the patient's right of choice exists whether the reasons for making that choice are rational, irrational, unknown or even non-existent. That his choice is contrary to what is to be expected of the vast majority of adults is only relevant if there are other reasons for doubting his capacity to decide.'

The UK Law Commission recommended that 'if a patient is incapacitated, and subject to other proposals in … this paper, a clearly established anticipatory decision should be as effective as the contemporaneous decision of the patient would be in the circumstances to which it is applicable.' In medical consent legislation in Ontario, Canada, if a person is deciding for another person who is not possessed with the legal capacity, then they must know that other person's wish 'expressed while capable and after attaining 16 years of age'; the decision maker 'shall take into consideration (a) the values and beliefs that the person knows the incapable person held while capable and (b) any wishes expressed by the incapable person.'

The question of the weight to be given to the concerns of relatives in deciding issues of consent for an incompetent patient was addressed in Re T. They have no legal right to make decision for a competent adult patient but their concerns have an important moral value when the issue of competence arises. The court adjudged it prudent to contact relatives to ascertain whether the patient has stated a prior refusal and whether the patient's views had changed subsequently.

The result of the necessary court intervention in the Irish Ward case (1995) was unsatisfactory. In that case, the High and Supreme Courts declared that the withdrawal of nutrition and hydration delivered by way of gastrostomy tube was lawful. The healthcare provider and institution looking after the ward had opposed the family's application. Despite calls on the relevant medical, legal and other professions for guidelines and clarification, no informative guidelines have since been issued by the Medical Council or other professional body nor has the issue been properly or openly debated. The Powers of Attorney Act 1996, which permitted a person to appoint another individual to have legally binding decision-making powers on his behalf, did not include healthcare provider decisions. It does however include 'personal care decisions' which may impinge on healthcare provider: where and with whom the person should live, whom he or she should see and not see, what training or rehabilitation he or she should get, diet and dress, inspection of personal papers, housing, social welfare, etc.

Article 8 of the European Convention on Human Rights sets out that 'everyone has the right to respect for his or her private and family life', and that 'there shall be no interference by a public authority with the exercise of this right except such as in accordance with the law'. When healthcare decisions and human life are being considered, there must be a clarity of understanding as to what is meant by value of human life, what constitutes basic care as opposed to medical treatment, the difference between chronic and terminal illness, and the medical criteria for intervention and withdrawal of treatment.

The withdrawal of treatment is a very difficult and emotive issue. It requires a proper understanding and assessment of medical futility, burden, and proportionality. Criteria must be set down in advance of situations where a patient requests withholding or withdrawal of treatment, resulting in death of that patient. Careful tests must be carried out as to the ethical and legal validity of such a request where it is made by a person other than the patient in circumstances where the patient is legally incompetent. Recourse to courts of law will be necessary where there is a conflict of opinion between those who state that they are acting on behalf of, or in the best interests of, the patient. When questions of 'rights' arise, it is necessary to examine the exact nature of the right to be vindicated. Does the 'right to die' mean: the right to be allowed die, the right to choose to die with dignity, the right to choose to be killed or the right to commit suicide? Does society have a proper and legitimate interest in protecting the right to life of all its members? Do citizens not also have to consider their duties to other members of society when asserting their 'right to die'?

Such 'right to die' decisions are of course the extreme examples of patient autonomy and consent in healthcare decisions. The conflicts that arise in such situations and the highly charged emotions provoked help to focus analysis of the issues. However, the autonomy of patients in the more mundane situations of consent to 'ordinary' medical intervention on an everyday basis should not be overlooked. There has been a fundamental shift in the healthcare provider-patient relationship and whilst it remains a relationship based on an inherent inequality, the era of medical paternalism has gone. Society now struggles with the problem of how to define and enhance patient autonomy without losing the trusting aspects so necessary and desirable in the relationship.

Conclusion

With increasing medical litigation and a striving for increased participation by patients in their healthcare decisions, the concept of autonomy and the areas of treatment consent and refusal are now a major legal battlefield, often to the detriment of the healthcare provider-patient relationship. An over-legalisation of patient consent or of the healthcare provider-patient relationship in general is not desirable. The patient has the right to know about his health and proposed interventions, to self-empowerment, to receive proper communications, and to litigate where appropriate. However, the patient also has the right to healthcare in a trusting relationship. The healthcare provider has the right to be trusted, the privilege of self-regulation and the obligation to continue professional education and undertake clinical audit and to communicate properly with patients. But he also has the right to defend reputation when impugned and the right to practice the art and science of caring in a trusting relationship.

The growing debate on the concept of patient autonomy is a healthy one. Although true patient autonomy may be a myth rather than a reality, that does not diminish in any way the respective rights and duties, safeguards and protections for both patient and healthcare provider. The future of healthcare and of the healthcare-patient relationship depends on the recognition of these mutual rights and duties both in law and medical ethics.

CHAPTER SIX

Ethics in Psychiatry

Marcus Webb

Introduction

The term 'psychiatry' refers to the medical treatment of the mind. Psychiatrists train first in medicine and then specialise in learning about and treating mental disorders. A senior English psychiatrist, Michael Shepherd, wrote about modern (British) psychiatry: 'at its core is an adherence to the principals of scientific enquiry in clinical and basic research, with due acknowledgement of the role played by social and psychological investigation as well as by the natural sciences.'[1] I think I need to explore these statements a little further in order to set the scene for discussion of some of the outstanding ethical issues in psychiatry.

Trust

Although the modern emphasis is on achieving near equality in the therapeutic relationship, many psychiatrists still would like to function with the old-fashioned medical, even Hippocratic values. The patient is the centre of medical attention: trust between patient and doctor is an important element in their interactions, and for good reasons.

Identifying the Abnormal

First, in psychiatry we are trying to sort out disorders of the highest human attainments: thoughts, memories, perceptions, language, attention, and emotions. There are no clear boundaries between what society calls normal in these areas and what it judges to be abnormal. A patient with schizophrenia may say that God is talking to him, but so may a devout person who does not suffer from schizophrenia. A bereaved wife may say she sees her dead husband coming in the front door, but she has no other distorted perceptions to suggest mental illness. Again, many delinquents and criminals demonstrate annoying or appalling antisocial behaviour, but social non-conformity alone must never be taken as the sole criterion of psychiatric disorder.[2] The political abuse of psychiatry that occurred in the Soviet Union in recent decades was one serious outcome of such a process.

Then there is the difficulty in deciding how anxious an individual must be before he is diagnosed as having an anxiety disorder. How depressed and for how long before he is judged to suffer a major depression? Useful psychological rating scales have been devised to assess severity of disordered mood, for example, but subjective judgement on the part of the professional raters still plays an important part.

New Technology
Second, the remarkable developments of medical technology of the last fifty years – and there has been amazing progress in the neurosciences – have not yet made their impact on everyday psychiatric assessments and treatments to the extent to which they have in clinical medicine. This means that psychiatrists cannot be, even if they wished to be, technologists relying on laboratory tests for diagnosis and offering the consumer a choice of procedures, but they need to engage their patients in a joint effort to achieve recovery.

Causes of mental disorders
Third, the absolute causes of mental disorders have not been determined in many cases, although we can frequently point to biological, psychological and social antecedents. Psychiatrists, who are part of, as well as observers of, the wider society, but who also have a scientific training, must seek widely to understand their patients' disorders and come to informed guesses, based on their knowledge and experience.

A great debate has always existed as to how far mind disorders are basically brain disorders. An individual thinking about his life may only contribute a small amount to the development and progress of his diabetes or high blood pressure, but mental disorders are likely to be the result of psychological processes as much as having a basic physical abnormality of the brain. Having said this, there is no doubt that subtle biochemical and electrical activities underlie our thinking, perception, memories, and emotional life. Also, to complicate matters further, the psychological meaning of our thoughts may trigger further physical changes – just consider the bodily changes accompanying embarrassing thoughts, exciting ideas, or fear.

People are further greatly influenced by the family, social and cultural circumstances in which they grow up and exist. Take for example a child growing up in a violent, alcoholic, dysfunctional family or as a refugee in a foreign country: such social factors make an important impact on how people view themselves, their self esteem, their reactions to others and their subsequent responses to stress. Such circumstances are well known to predispose to mental disorders.

Mind, brain, and body are not then the separate entities we often imagine them to be, and no one psychologist, sociologist, or biologist has a monopoly of knowledge that can unravel the very complex origins of the mental disorders. To illustrate this point further, a psychologist may view a patient with depression as experiencing the awakened loss of his mother in childhood. A social interpretation may be that he is reacting to constricting and demeaning social circumstances of unemployment and poverty, while a biological psychiatrist might highlight genetic predisposition to depression and excessive release of a chemical cortisol into the bloodstream, which is not controlled by normal brain mechanisms. They may all be correct, and it is the job of the psychiatrist to decide, on limited evidence, and without an unequivocal explanatory model for guidance, which of these paths it would be most beneficial to pursue and to try to correct.

We can now fairly reliably make diagnoses such as major depression, obsessive compulsive disorder, anorexia nervosa, bipolar disorder, schizophrenia and so on, because of internationally agreed descriptions of the disorders,[3,4] but their absolute causes remain in dispute. Where there is such doubt ethical issues are bound to arise. Is it ethical to involve a patient in extensive and expensive sessions of psychotherapy to help him to come to terms with a disastrous childhood if his depression is characterised by a chemical imbalance that can be efficiently removed by antidepressant medication in a much shorter time? On the contrary, is it appropriate to use an antidepressant drug that sometimes has troublesome side effects, when cognitive psychotherapy gives understanding about an underlying faulty self-appraisal by the patient, resulting in a healthier future without relapse? Opinions on individual cases inevitably differ where precise causes remain uncertain. Again, a wider social question, is it ethically necessary for the psychiatrist, who sees the serious mental results of poor social conditions, to launch public campaigns for a more equitable society, or is it sufficient that he keep his head down and do his best for his individual patients and their families? Again, should he work harder to dispel the disabling stigma with which our society still views mental disorders, despite their frequency in the general population?

These are the sort of questions doctors have always had to face where the best available answer has to be arrived at with incomplete evidence for guidance. Psychiatrists have to tolerate uncertainty in their efforts to do their best for their patient. Trust is a necessary ingredient, but the Hippocratic tradition is no longer a sufficient basis on which to conduct psychiatric practice.

Development of Ethical Thinking in Psychiatry

Ethical issues in psychiatry were until recent decades seen as no different from those of general medical treatments.[5] The doctor respected his patient, tried to do his best for him, and maintained strict confidentiality. This sufficed for a private, office-type of practice, and perhaps still can do so. The individual patient who has the capacity to decide for himself consults his chosen doctor and can stop doing so if he wishes.

But various features of the practice of psychiatry demanded special attention. For one hundred years, until the latter decades of this century, very many patients were looked after in large, often forbidding and poorly funded institutions. Most patients were sent to the asylums involuntarily. Effective treatments hardly existed. Even enlightened and learned doctors such as Connolly Norman of the Richmond Asylum and Richard Leeper of St Patrick's Hospital could do little more than contain disturbed behaviour in a humane manner, encourage good nutrition and physical activity, and wait and hope for spontaneous improvement.

Then earlier concepts[6] of trying to avoid the demoralising and debasing effects of institutional life by managing patients in smaller, more domestic settings in the community, and indeed in their own homes, were brought back. Treatments with remarkable drugs became available in the 1950s, and day care was introduced. Specific psychological and social theories heralded new treatments and new therapists: psychologists, social workers and occupational therapists joined nurses and doctors in multi-disciplinary teams which offered combined care and treatment. The patient's family was more often directly included in assessment and management. And so here we are at the end of twentieth century with an array of treatment approaches and care settings which did not exist fifty years ago.

Ethical issues have arisen in all of these changed practices, but in fact are accentuated by the great shift in society's attitude towards the autonomy of the individual, as promulgated in the last century by Mill[8] and as developed in the twentieth century by the human rights movement.[9] Previously patients were placed in asylums, it appeared, for the supposed benefit of the wider community as much as for the care of the individual patient. Now much more stringent mental health laws are being introduced to safeguard the individual's autonomy, although not always, it has to be said, with the expected benefits for the patient's health. A tension exists particularly poignantly in psychiatry, and it is being played out at the present time, between the medical paternalism of the past and the modern concept of the autonomy of the individual. I hope to illustrate this tension in discussing confidentiality, involuntary treatment, informed consent, and the problems posed by the personality disordered, in the remaining sections of this paper.

Confidentiality

Communication is a catch cry of modern life. In psychiatry, the multidisciplinary team provides broadly based care for the individual. But this means that information about the patient must be shared between the professional members of the team. Information follows patients around the community facilities, from outpatient clinic to day hospital care: from the inpatient unit to the high support hostel to the rehabilitation centre. Some patients feel very keenly this spread of knowledge about their very personal concerns. If the patient can give informed consent to this style of care there is no great ethical issue, but consent may at times be presumed rather than sought directly when the conviction of staff is that this form of care is the very best available for the patient. If the patient clearly states his unwillingness to have such personal information shared with others, than the doctor would normally respect his wish.

It is now generally accepted that a patient's confidence may be broken in very few, well defined situations:[10] when ordered by a judge in a court of law, when necessary to protect the interest of the patient, to protect the welfare of the wider society, and to safeguard another individual. I leave aside third party payment situations that are causing increasing concern. We are very unhappy frequently that our case notes and memories of patients should be required by law to be made available in court without our patient's permission, and there is no doubt that such legal activities have eroded trust between doctor and patient. Difficult decisions have to be faced at times when others are in danger: we learn, for example, that our patient, an airline pilot, has become an unreliable alcoholic, a medical colleague has become addicted to drugs, a husband is known to suffer from a sexually transmitted disease, but will not tell his wife, or a paranoid patient harbours aggressive intentions towards another person. The well-known Tarasoff case in Berkeley, California, established legal principle in just such a case: the psychiatrist told the police but not the victim when the patient threatened to kill his ex-girlfriend. Obviously, one tries to persuade the patient to allow the disclosure or to make it himself, but failing this, one may have a duty of care to break the confidence of the patient and warn the potential victim.

Issues of Consent and Involuntary Treatment

1. Consent:

Some patients are admitted unconscious or in a delirious state to general hospitals. The doctor's duty of care – to do the best he can for his patient – ensures that he treats this person to the best of his ability and with respect for the patient's dignity, even though the patient cannot give his consent. Such paternalism indeed used to be more widely applied throughout medicine. Patients trusted their doctor to do their best for them and followed his advice, and the doctor accepted this responsibility. This relationship was built into the Hippocratic tradition. Psychiatrists face an allied problem when a patient's mental capacity is insufficient to give or to withhold valid consent to be treated. Consider a deluded, a mentally handicapped, or a demented individual who lacks capacity to judge whether he should be treated. In such situations, the doctor will normally seek consent from a relative of his patient. More elaborate legal strategies to provide satisfactory decisions on behalf of patients who lack capacity include guardianship, care orders and wardship of court. Each of these strategies has limitations, and observers are now suggesting that the patient when well, or a judicial process when necessary, should appoint an independent advocate for the patient who will give an unbiased view on the acceptability of a proposed course of action. In Northern Ireland and in the Netherlands, this system, although cumbersome, is thought to be working well. It may in time provide welcome support for seeking improved resources in psychiatry, in addition.

2. Involuntary admission:

Deluded patients usually do not appreciate that they are unwell, but may object to being brought into hospital and treated. Involuntary admissions constitute about ten per cent of admissions to psychiatric hospitals in Ireland at the present time. The large majority of patients therefore enter hospital voluntarily. Virtually every country enacts legislation to enable seriously mentally ill patients to be admitted to hospitals against their will if they pose a danger to themselves or to others. In most countries, patients also may be so admitted if their health is seriously deteriorating for want of suitable care and treatment.

The concept here is that individuals have a right to their autonomy which cannot be readily set aside, but they also have a right to be treated when they are ill, even when they do not appreciate their need.

Thus, patients, who are so depressed that they are seriously considering suicide, yet refuse treatment, may be admitted on a detention order. Again, the very occasional patient who may respond to delusions – which are false beliefs – or to auditory hallucinations, or by being aggressive to others, may be admitted involuntarily. Similarly people who are neglecting themselves, living in increasingly squalid conditions, or are seriously vulnerable in society by virtue of their mental illness may be admitted against their will.

This process is not a task psychiatrists relish: it can be a harrowing and unpleasant experience for all concerned, and only sometime later when the patient recovers is the humane value of appropriate mental health laws fully appreciated.

To deprive someone of their liberty is an extremely serious matter and, of course, it must be carried out under strict conditions prescribed by law.[11] The procedure is that someone in the community, usually a close relative, makes an application to a hospital on the appropriate form. A doctor who has no connection with the hospital, usually the patient's general practitioner, must examine the patient and then if he thinks the individual suffers from mental illness and needs hospital care he may make a medical recommendation on part 2 of the form. The consultant psychiatrist then considers the application and recommendation and, if he agrees, he signs the reception order and it becomes a legal document enabling the admission. Thus, there are safeguards against wrongful admission. Also, the patient may appeal against involuntary admission to the Minister for Health, the CEO of the Health Board, the Inspector of Mental Hospitals, or the President of the High Court. Further limits and conditions apply to care in hospitals.

A moral issue for our society in Ireland exists today in that the Mental Treatment Act 1945 has not been replaced for over fifty years. During these decades, there have been tremendous social changes and medical advances. A new act with further safeguards for patients in line with modern concepts of autonomy and human rights has been promised since the publication of a Green Paper in 1992,[7] and has only recently been published. Mental health in our country does not carry high political priority. In Northern Ireland, there have been two new mental health acts since the 1940s and a further revision is planned.

The ethical basis of admitting and treating people against their will has been challenged, understandably, but most notably by certain psychiatrists. Dr Thomas Szasz, a New York professor of psychiatry, and incidentally a friend of our late and much lamented Trinity colleague Dr Petr Skrabanek, has gone further and has denied the existence of mental illness. In his book, *The myth of mental illness,* he argues that mental disorders are not illnesses in the sense of medical diseases, and that people must be held responsible for their own behaviour.[12] He is consistent at least in that he has written that if people misbehave they should be brought before a court of law and punished if they are found guilty, but they should not be forced into hospital and given treatment against their will. Also, he says that it is a person's right to commit suicide if he so wishes and a diagnosis of a

depressive illness is of no consequence. Coercion and deprivation of liberty in the name of treatment is, in his view, a greater
catastrophe.

To the practising psychiatrist dealing with seriously disordered patients and to the suffering relatives and friends, the contributions of Dr Szasz and others along these lines seem to be
dangerous academic polemic, but there is no doubt that his
views have forced people to think carefully about these issues
and to take very seriously indeed the deprivation of others'
liberty. In fact, Szasz recognises, as did Mill in the nineteenth
century, that children need to be subject to special care and con-
trols and be relieved of certain responsibilities by the State. He
differs from most people in that he denies that adults may suffer
from mental disorders which may put them in as much need of
special care and control as children, or that they should therefore on occasions be relieved of certain responsibilities. The
American courts, however, have taken the views of Szasz almost
to their limits. It is extremely difficult to enforce hospitalisation
and treatment in some States, and mental disorder is again a
daily spectacle in all its tragedy on the streets. The human rights
pendulum has swung.

Recent Legal Decisions
Consider again the mentally handicapped or demented individual who lacks capacity to decide if he should be admitted to hospital. Many such patients are brought to the wards informally
by relatives. In December 1997 the Court of Appeal in the UK
ruled that an autistic and profoundly retarded patient who did
not have the capacity to decide on his own care should be on a
detention order in hospital, and that he should not be just maintained there informally as he did not actively refuse to stay.[13]
This decision sent shock waves through the healthcare system,
as there were many thousands of such patients in hospitals and
indeed nursing homes throughout the country in just such circumstances. Those detained under the Mental Health Act would
have to increase from around 13,000 to 35,000, with all the atten-

dant problems. A parliamentary committee is examining the issue to find a way around the legal and ethical tangle, and it may well come up with a new procedure, separate from psychiatric reception orders. Similar considerations need to be undertaken in managing demented patients. A positive result has been the realisation that formal methods of measuring incapacity need to be devised.

Another recent case in the UK found that a mentally handicapped patient detained under the Mental Health Act 1983, because of behavioural disturbances, was yet competent to refuse haemodialysis to save her life.[14] In this instance the patient was found by the court to be able to comprehend and retain information about the proposed treatment, was able to understand the information, and she had the capacity to weigh such information in the balance in order to reach a choice. The court ordered that she should not be forced to undergo haemodialysis and, presumably, she died.

Our 1945 Act allows treatment to be given to a detained patient in hospital without his consent. In many states of the USA, consent to treatment, other than emergency treatment, is required before even medication may be administered to patients who are detained. The bizarre situation thus is developing whereby hospitals are again becoming simply custodial institutions, somewhat like ancient mad houses. The law detains patients but psychiatrists are not allowed to give more than emergency treatment if the patient refuses. Dr Alan Stone, former President of the American Psychiatric Association, reports that the courts in the USA have found that emergency treatment only applies to patients being dangerous and does not cover sufficient treatment to ensure recovery from psychosis.[15] This appears to many to be a denial of the patients' rights to be treated in overweening pursuit of their right to make autonomous decisions. Unfortunately, psychiatrists in large numbers are abandoning the seriously mentally ill in the public health service in the USA under these conditions, for a less impossible life looking after the less severely ill and the 'worried well' who are present in many private, office-style settings. Presumably, this action is an expression of the doctors' own human rights. In the UK, the issue of treatment of detained patients is handled somewhat better in that a second opinion by a registered psychiatrist may allow longer treatment to be given. However, the law and the human rights movement sometimes move in mysterious ways. In a celebrated public appeal in the United Kingdom a consultant surgeon asked how the law and medical ethics have insisted that his son with schizophrenia may continue to live in squalor in a cave, apparently in deference to the boy's stated wishes, but in defiance of his need to be treated.

In Australia, where community psychiatry has been comparatively well funded, patients may now be required by law to take medication while living in the community, thus enabling them to stay well and autonomous in other ways. This does seem a more humane and far preferable approach but it overrides a patient's refusal and is not in fact trouble-free. My worry is that most things that happen in the United States come here about twenty years later and I just hope that our society will retain a reasonable balance between need for treatment and right to autonomy. I will thankfully no longer be in practice if patients are to be allowed in this country to 'rot with their rights on' as one observer called this process.[16] Unfortunately, I could well by then qualify as a demented patient, and I hope humanity will remain in relation to ethical choices in our country.

Personality Disorder
Finally, I want to talk about some problems presented to psychiatry by individuals with personality disorder. These problems are highlighted nowadays because of the increasing accessibility of psychiatric treatment and modern concepts of care.

If you think for a moment about your relatives, friends and even enemies, you will be well aware that personal characteristics vary remarkably. Some are more anxious, some more perfectionists, some more suspicious, others more histrionic and dramatic than the rest and others are even more antisocial. It is apparent that individuals with the more extreme characteristics tend to cause problems, particularly in their relationships with others, for themselves and sometimes for their fellow men and women. Some of those who suffer or who come into conflict with others we may refer to as having personality disorders. They do not suffer from psychotic or delusional illnesses. They are not mentally handicapped, demented, persistently depressed or suffer from any of the broad groups of mental illness which have been categorised by psychiatrists over time. They understand how society expects them to behave, and, in ordinary terms, they can control what they do. People with personality disorders may indeed complain of depression or anxiety briefly but there is no consistency to the syndromes despite a pattern of disrupted relationships. They may abuse alcohol or other drugs but unless they become dependent on these drugs, such abuse tends to be sporadic rather than compulsive.

Severe Personality Disorders
It is in fact very difficult to change patterns of behaviour where they are not part of an illness. The influences that have contributed to such abnormal behaviour have persisted for years and it would be arrogant for psychiatrists to pretend that several hours of discussion with such individuals could change their lives. Critical journalists,[17] on the other hand, often write that if only psychiatrists would follow this or that system of psychotherapy their severely personality disordered patients would remarkably transform their patterns of thought and behaviour. Would that therapy were so simple. Nowadays people with personality disorders may present to practitioners or hospitals looking for help, often because of self-injury or overdose. In cases of antisocial personality, they may be brought for help to the hospital by despairing relatives, or may be seen in prison by forensic psychiatrists.

There are now very many fewer hospital beds than there were even twenty years ago. Inevitably, those who are in these beds are the most seriously ill and it is easy to appreciate that men and women with antisocial personality cannot be managed effectively in the smaller, more open general hospital psychiatric units where most patients are now admitted. Disturbed behaviour cannot be 'absorbed' in such small units as it used to be in the larger hospitals. Also, society, and particularly that element which tends toward antisocial behaviour, is becoming more aggressive and violent. It is absolutely unacceptable that a few individuals with antisocial personality should be allowed to disturb the treatment of other patients, and even to put their lives in danger.

Far from seeking to have such individuals admitted involuntarily, psychiatrists generally try to manage them as out patients, but with great difficulty. These patients are inconsistent in attending for appointments: they are impulsive and could indeed harm themselves if not admitted in crisis. They do suffer and they do make other people suffer. The question constantly arises these days whether or not the psychiatric services should try to look after them. There are many of these patients who hit the tabloid headlines: 'Hospital discharges suicidal patient', 'My daughter is denied psychiatric treatment', and so on.

This is an ethical issue for our time, highlighted by the increasing, ready violence of our society. Psychiatrists are ambivalent: on the one hand the behaviour, relationships, attitudes, conscience structures of these individuals are undoubtedly abnormal. Surely, psychiatrists have knowledge and responsibilities in these areas. On the other hand, we have no suitable facilities or effective treatments. We can sedate people with antisocial personality, try to provide consistent psychological boundaries, but these have only short-term effects and do not induce actual change. Psychiatrists on the right wing say these people can take their own decisions, we can't treat them effectively and so we should not use up valuable resources, and upset other patients by trying to do so. Psychiatrists on the left wing point out that the history of medicine is full of examples of disorders which were at one time not effectively treated: if we study them and try new treatment methods, sooner or later something will come up. The issue has been highlighted recently in the UK where the Home Secretary has declared the government's intention to detain certain aggressive antisocial personalities, e.g. dangerous psychopaths, paedophiles, indefinitely, even when they have completed their prison sentence, or even when they have not committed a crime.[18] Of great concern also is the apparent intention to detain such individuals in hospitals, although this is opposed by the Royal College of Psychiatrists which has stated that psychiatrists are not jailers and they have no effective treatment for severely personality disordered individuals.[19] This is a major issue for psychiatry at the turn of the millennium. It is difficult to know if this is a special case or whether the human rights pendulum is swinging back.

Conclusion

I pointed out earlier that medical practice has always meant making informed choices where there are few certainties. There is already an explosion of knowledge in the neurosciences, which will increasingly aid our treatment choices in psychiatry. But the individual's life history and social circumstances will surely demand of psychiatry that the technologist will never entirely replace the medical practitioner. Difficult clinical and ethical decisions are likely to continue to be the stuff of psychiatric practice. The Declaration of Hawaii advises us to continue to treat our patients with solicitude and respect, and to the best of our ability and knowledge. Thomas Szasz berates us for coercing people we believe are mentally ill and we must heed the final words of his book, *Cruel Compassion:*[20] 'all history teaches us to beware of benefactors who deprive their beneficiaries of liberty.' We should continue to try to achieve trust between our patients and ourselves and to understand more about the nature of mental disorders.

CHAPTER SEVEN

Legislating the Right to Die: Perspectives and Prescriptions

Patrick Hanafin

'Authorities, sacred and secular, do not care for the thought; they do not want you to be dead. Except, perhaps, as a martyr, and even this they have their doubts about.' (Ricks, *Beckett's Dying Words*, p. 1)

Introduction

Fintan O'Toole, writing recently in the wake of Archbishop Desmond Connell's intervention in the debate on *in vitro* fertilisation, concluded that: 'We are at a key moment in Irish history when an old set of values has been destroyed and a new one has not yet been developed.' (O'Toole, 'Archbishop's insensitivity arises from ignorance', *Irish Times*, 5 March 1999, p 8) This reflects the centrality of bioethical questions in the debate over Irish societal values. As in other areas of biomedical ethics, the area of death and dying reflects this conflict between competing notions of societal identity. For too long individual self-determination in the area of biomedical ethics has been subordinated to an ideal conception of the societal good based on communal and conservative values. The history of the struggle for reproductive freedom in Ireland bears ample testimony to this phenomenon. I attempt here to investigate the manner in which medicine, law and pressure groups in their construction of treatment withdrawal reflect broader cultural conflict over the redefinition of Irish citizenship.

The body has been and continues to be a controversial site of contestation over notions of value, identity and citizenship in Irish law. The conservative discourse around the body in the opening decades of the Irish State was to have profound repercussions for the ability of the individual to control her own body. Thus, elite discourses of politics, law, medicine and the church created a climate in which control of the individual body was a priority. While the overarching notion of Irish national identity has been transformed, and legal change in the area of biomedical dilemmas is being discussed if not effected, what persists is a basic split in the notion of how the body is to be envisioned in Irish society and as a corollary, the manner in which Irish society is to be visualised.

The decision in *Re A Ward of Court* gave legal recognition to the chronically ill patient's right to die naturally. However, this temporary resolution of the issue is by no means definitive and has merely set the tone for the debate over the legal and ethical regulation of death and dying which will continue into the next century. The reaction to the decision both at the level of legal argument and in public debate has opened up a cleavage in Irish society only too familiar after three decades of intensive debate over other bioethical issues. The initial reaction from the medical profession has not been accepting of the decision, revealing a position that is antithetical to the introduction of policy that would allow for the legalisation of treatment withdrawal. The decision itself raises its own questions as to the exact boundaries of treatment withdrawal.

Biomedical discourse around death and dying is part of a wider societal antipathy to dying, and in particular, a societal dread of death, of losing the battle against disease, of having one's borders penetrated by contaminating disease. Likewise at the societal level, Ireland has until quite recently been a hermetically sealed society in relation to questions of bioethical controversy. Contraception and abortion were all seen in certain quarters as part of the contaminating influence of alien cultures and were to be repelled through a public policy of criminalisation of individual choice. Only in the past thirty years has this paradigm been challenged and a more heterogeneous society has begun to emerge. However, this does not mean that there is a societal consensus on all issues of bioethical controversy. For each step forward in terms of the recognition of individual rights in this area, there is a concomitant step backwards due to the lack of constructive public policy developments in this area. Court victories in many cases do not lead to greater access to the means of exercising these rights in practice. As Ailbhe Smyth has put it: 'there are indeed many ways in which the everyday realities of Irish life give the lie to the shiny image of progress and modernism'. (Smyth, 'And Nobody was any the Wiser' in *Sexual Politics and the European Union*, p. 113) The question of death and dying is the latest area of bioethical controversy that continues this peculiar pattern of change and stasis.

The Professional Regulation of Death
Society endeavours to alleviate the dread of death by medicalising the dying process, and in so doing, attempts to persuade itself that death has been conquered by technology. By placing a technological overlay on the dying process, one is creating a situation where it is impossible to die. In the modern era, increasing technological complexity allows us to keep patients in a state of living death raising the inevitable ethical and legal questions of when does life end and when can we intervene to terminate the lives of those in such a condition. The question of who decides such questions and how they do so has become an increasingly contentious question for doctors, lawyers, patients and politicians alike. In Gidden's words:

'Death has become a technical matter, its assessment removed into the hands of the medical profession; what death is becomes a matter of deciding at what point a person should be treated as having died, in respect of the cessation of various types of bodily function. Death remains the great extrinsic factor of human existence ... Death becomes a point zero: it is nothing more or less than the moment at which human control over human existence finds an outer limit.' (Giddens, *Modernity and Self-Identity*, p. 161)

As a result, the question of deciding when one should die has been taken out of the hands of the dying and placed in the institutional framework of the medical and legal professions. As Beck has observed: 'What is considered and recognised socially as "life" and "death" becomes contingent in and through the work of medical people themselves. It must be redetermined with all the foreseeable implications – and against the background and on the foundation of circumstances, problems and criteria produced by medicine and biology.' (Beck, *Risk Society*, p. 210) This death has brought in its wake the increased interest of the legal profession. Daniel Callahan notes that in abandoning the collective idea of a common destiny, we have robbed death of its cultural significance and have been unable to find an enduring replacement. Thus, he claims:

'We do not have the shared sense of destiny ... We have tried, to be sure, to find substitutes, but in each case they turn out to be ways of better mastering and controlling death, not of finding a common way to seek and share its meaning and accept its inevitability.' (Callahan, *The Troubled Dream of Life*, p. 225)

He sees a need to re-evaluate the medical interpretation of death, to divest ourselves of what he terms 'technological monism', by which he means: 'the tendency to erase the difference between human action as a cause of what happens in the world, and independent, natural biological processes, those old-fashioned causes of disease and death'. (Callahan, *The Troubled Dream of Life*, p. 67) It is in this idea of 'technological monism' that we can begin to see the reason why law has become increasingly involved in the treatment of the dying. The move from seeing nature as the culpable party in the death of the individual to seeing the individual medical professional as culpable, has inevitably brought law, with its ideas of fault and responsibility, into the scenario. The dying patient, unable to die as a result of the technological imperative in modernist medicine, must obtain the approval of the law to embark on such a course. This modernist conception of the dying patient is redolent of Arthur Frank's analysis of the chronically ill patient:

'As patients, these folk accumulate entries on medical charts

... the chart becomes the official story of the illness ... The story told by the physician becomes the one against which [other narratives] are ultimately judged true or false, useful or not ... I understand this obligation of seeking medical care as a narrative surrender and mark it as the central moment in modernist illness experience.' (Frank, *The Wounded Storyteller*, p. 6)

The notion of 'narrative surrender' is a familiar one in the history of medico-legal controversies in Ireland. The individual's narrative is rarely heard. Instead, the patient is constructed through legal and medical narratives. Thus in cases like *McGee v Attorney-General* and *Attorney-General v X*, the individual patient is presented as a problem to be solved, the real voice behind the case is rarely heard. This was made even more clear in the case of *Re A Ward of Court* where the patient was literally voiceless. In the absence of living will legislation or even a living will, the patient was presented through the narratives of her relatives, the judiciary and of sundry medical and legal professionals. The individual's access to his own death had now to be secured through the instrumentality of legal professionals making death an even more impersonal and remote experience. The way in which the law and policy-makers deal with such issues is informed by various ethical views on life and death, thus further clouding the issue.

In this sense, ethical discourse is never neutral. In other words, the apparently objective technical discourse of medicine reflects particular cultural and ethical values that belie this apparent assumption of objectivity. This can be seen in the statement issued by the Medical Council in the wake of the Ward case, which, couched in diplomatic terms, was nonetheless infused with particular assumptions about the position of the patient in ethical terms. In addition, the gnomic references to chronically ill patients in the Medical Council's latest ethical guidelines belie a particular far from objective view on such treatments. (Irish Medical Council, *A Guide to Ethical Conduct and to Fitness to Practise*, 1998, p. 38) This reflects Catherine

Waldby's thesis in which she argues that medical discourse translates notions of power and individual governance into societal reality:

'Biomedicine is a useful discourse of governance precisely because of its capacity to translate social relations into 'neutral' technical discourses ... This capacity enables it to intervene in detailed ways in a social field, to practise a micropolitics of the body and a macropolitics of the body politic, subsuming both domains of intervention under the flexible rhetoric of health. Biomedicine is able to articulate both domains because ... its representations of the body always involve the analogisation of the body to highly normative understandings of social order, and a reciprocal analogisation of the social order according to its normative representations of the body. This normative reciprocity allows biomedicine to readily conceptualise the relationship between particular bodies and its hierarchical, hygienic programme for social order. Its arsenal of technical and behavioural technologies helps it to reconcile particular bodily morphologies with the changing demands of that order.' (Waldby, *AIDS and the Body Politic*, p. 141)

The Legal Construction of Treatment Withdrawal

The typical trajectory in relation to securing the rights of the individual in areas of bioethical controversy in Ireland has been for the courts to derive a right based on constitutional principles, and then for a split or fissure to emerge in society over the issue, leading to government inaction and the inability of individuals to access that right in practice. In effect, the situation created could be seen as causing more problems than it solves.

Cass Sunstein has, in the context of the United States Supreme Court's intervention in areas of public controversy including bioethical disputes, argued for a minimalist model whereby the court takes a less aggressive role, leaving decisions to be made through a process of State legislative intervention after a period of public debate (Sunstein, 'The Right to Die', *The*

Yale Law Journal). Perhaps, he is being too pessimistic or indeed playing a strategic game in an era of a conservative court. In playing a more aggressive role in the area of recognition of individual liberty, the Supreme Court does, after all, put on the public agenda the question of individual rights in the bioethical arena.

This leads to greater deliberation in society on these questions, leading in many cases to legislative intervention following widespread consultation. At a more general level, the expansion of rights discourse marks a shift in societal views in relation to bodily autonomy. This is if one takes the problematic view that societal changes can be reflected at the level of legal discourse. Cass Sunstein has defined this process as law's 'expressive function' (Sunstein, *One Case at a Time*, p. 953). Law's 'expressive function' refers to the manner in which law expresses social and cultural values and encourages social norms to move in particular directions. However, the values which law expresses are not fixed for all time and may change as societal norms and values change. Thus, when society experiences a 'norm cascade' (Sunstein, *One Case at a Time*, p. 912), that is, a rapid shift towards new norms, such norm shifts may be expressed in legal discourse.

This however does not ignore the fact that certain groups in society will resist such changes. Similarly, in Ireland, over the past thirty years, in part through their recognition in constitutional rights discourse, a move to altered perceptions of cultural values has occurred in Ireland. On the symbolic level, this has expressed itself as a move from notions of control over the individual's ability to dispose with them as they wish to a less constricted notion of individual self-determination. On the practical level, strategies of resistance have been instantiated, which make it difficult for such rights to be exercised.

Thus, following the case of *Attorney-General v X*, abortion legislation has not yet been introduced but the government has begun a consultation process. Similarly, in the United Kingdom, following the case of *R. v Bourne* in 1939, thirty years elapsed before public policy caught up with legal reality, thus indicating the need for value shifts to evolve before controversial policy issues can be successfully tackled. After the decision in the McGee case 1973 it took another twenty years before widespread access to contraception was secured and it was not until 1997 that a national policy initiative in the area of fertility was introduced (Murphy-Lawless and McCarthy, 'Social Policy and Fertility Change in Ireland', *The European Journal of Women's Studies*).

The debate was initiated via pressure from judicial decisions and changing societal attitudes. Law expresses this shift; it does not necessarily cause it, but acts as a means of signalling a change in previously dominant societal attitudes, indicating the emergence of new values. As Berkovitch has noted in analysing the link between law and cultural values:

'Law can be conceived as a cultural product; like other such products, law embodies and expresses specific social ideologies through its assumptions about society and its various members ... At the same time, law also plays an active role. Through its discourse it reproduces and constitutes both the societal subjects and their interrelations ... Law reflects as well as reproduces social structures.' (Berkovitch, 'Motherhood as a National Mission: The Construction of Womanhood in the Legal Discourse in Israel', *Women's Studies International Forum*, p. 607)

The recognition of a right of the chronically ill patient to refuse artificial nutrition and hydration has undergone a similar trajectory: recognition of the legal and ethical dilemmas, a temporary solution by the Supreme Court and then the instantiation of strategies of resistance. This raises the question of constitutional fit. In other words, does the pronouncement by the Supreme Court on the existence of a right to pregnancy termination or a right to treatment withdrawal exist anywhere other than in the language of the court? Given the evidence of the past thirty years, it would appear that the translation of the right into a societal reality is fraught with difficulty, caused by barriers raised by powerful groups in society. These constitutional rights remain in abeyance due to the power of professional regulatory bodies to define these rights as unethical. Thus, we have witnessed the effective blocking of these rights in practice.

This raises questions about the legitimacy of constitutional decision-making in this area. Inevitably, it is for the legislature to engage in some form of deliberative decision-making in this area. This would involve a wide-ranging debate on the issue in order to come to some democratic decision on the issue. A consultative process leading to legislative reform, for example, would be an acceptable democratic means of resolving conflict in this area. The courts in Ireland have for too long been forced to act as pseudo-legislators, a role they have acknowledged and about which they have raised concerns. Thus, the late Justice Niall McCarthy in *Attorney-General v X* noted: 'It is not for the courts to programme society; that is partly, at least, the role of the legislature. The courts are not equipped to regulate these procedures.' ([1992] 1 IR 1, p. 83) More recently, in 1997, Justice O'Flaherty noted in relation to abortion: 'It is not the function of this court to supplement this governmental and legislative inertia by making orders so uncertain and fraught with difficulty.' This is not to lessen the positive transformative role that the court has played in reflecting changes in Irish society over the past thirty years. It is merely to point out that the reason the court has been forced to play such a role is due to governmental inaction in the area of healthcare and human rights.

In the case of *Re A Ward of Court* ([1995] 2 ILRM, p. 401) the person behind the appellation, Ward of Court, was a forty-five-year-old woman who at the age of twenty-two suffered irreversible brain damage during a minor surgical procedure under general anaesthetic. This left her in a near persistent vegetative state. She was kept alive since the mishap by means of artificial hydration and nutrition. The ward was unable to communicate. She had minimal capacity to recognise nursing staff and to react to strangers by showing signs of distress. She was able to follow people with her eyes in a reflex manner. Her family was of the opinion that it was in her 'best interests' that she be allowed to die naturally. The patient's family applied to the High Court for an order directing artificial nutrition and hydration to cease. The institution in which the ward resided objected to such an order, claiming that it was contrary to its ethical code and not in her 'best interests' that she be allowed to die naturally. Accordingly, the family applied to the High Court for an order directing artificial nutrition and hydration to cease, where Justice Lynch heard the application.

Justice Lynch was of the opinion that in the case of an incompetent, incurably ill patient, the healthcare provider in question may, subject to the acquiescence of the next-of-kin, lawfully withdraw life-sustaining medical treatment or refrain from providing such treatment. In this case, the healthcare providers objected to this withdrawal of treatment. Justice Lynch held that in such a case the test to be applied is whether it is in the 'best interests' of the patient that her life should be prolonged by artificial means. Justice Lynch also took into account what would be the patient's own wishes if she could be granted a momentary lucid period. The judge concluded that the courts in such cases should 'approach the matter from the standpoint of a prudent, good and loving parent in deciding what course should be adopted.' ([1995] 2 ILRM 401, p. 419)

The dying patient thus became a pawn in a game between two competing sets of interests. The law as arbiter imposed the compromise principle of best interests that did not pertain to the best interest of the actual patient but of the best interests of the patient as mediated via the medico-legal gaze. In the High Court, the invisibility of this particular patient was encapsulated in the judge's conclusion that the courts in such cases should 'approach the matter from the standpoint of a prudent, good and loving parent in deciding what course should be adopted', thus adding a paternalistic twist to the decision and further infantalising the ward.

Justice Lynch, while maintaining that the 'acid test' was the best interests test, also stated that he could take into account the wards' wishes 'if she could be granted a momentary lucid and articulate period in which to express them'. ([1995] 2 ILRM 401, p. 418-19) This mingling of the best interests and substituted judgement test is a much less sophisticated version of the hybrid model adopted by some courts in the United States to overcome some of the problems involved with the substituted judgement test. Thus, in the New Jersey Supreme Court decision in *In Re Conroy* (486 A. 2d 1209 [1985]), the court adopted a three stage test which combined elements of both the substituted judgement and best interests tests. This was a case where the patient had not made an advance directive. The court held that in the first stage of the test the substituted judgement test should be applied. However, if there was not enough evidence of the patient's wishes in this regard, the decision-maker should then proceed to decide on the basis of the best interests test. At this stage, the decision-maker could choose from one of two versions of the best interests test. If one decided on the basis of the limited-objective test, then there would have to be some evidence of the patient's past wishes but not enough to satisfy the substituted judgement test. Alternatively, one could decide on the basis of the pure-objective test, where there is no evidence at all of the patient's wishes in this area.

As one commentator has noted with regard to the court's approach in *In Re Conroy:*

'Rather than viewing the "subjective" and "best interests" tests as polar opposites ... envisions them as points on a continuum in which the "subjective" standard is but a particularised application of the "best interests" standard, the meaning of which comes from the patient's own subjective preferences.' (Meisel, *The Right to Die*, p. 279)

This test was to be confined to patients in a similar fact situation, namely, an elderly nursing home resident, suffering from serious mental and physical impairment (in this case Alzheimer's and diabetes) and who will probably die within one year even with the treatment. She was not PVS but was hardly conscious. The court found that the burdens of continued treatment did not outweigh the benefits of continuing the treatment and the court refused to order discontinuation of treatment. The types of burdens that are typically taken into account in such cases are pain, indignity, and quality of life. In Conroy, the burden that was given greatest consideration was pain. Consequently, under both limbs of the Conroy objective test it will be quite difficult to justify treatment withdrawal in many cases. On the one hand, this provides a safeguard in cases such as the elderly Alzheimer's patient. On the other hand, from the point of view of a patient wishing to refuse continued treatment in such circumstances, the overemphasis on the criterion of pain in arriving at a decision requires, as Meisel has argued:

'that treatment is administered even when it accomplishes little or nothing more than prolonging the process of dying … Some patients experience no actual pain because they are not suffering from a painful terminal illness, are in a persistent vegetative state, or are receiving strong analgesic medications. Even if the patient is able to experience pain, the judicious use of analgesic medications can usually control it to the extent to which a patient perceives pain may be difficult even if the patient is not comatose. Thus, pain should not be the sole, or even the central, criterion in determining the burdens that treatment imposes.' (Meisel, *The Right to Die*, pp 291-2)

In subsequent cases, the New Jersey Supreme Court has held that in relation to patients in a persistent vegetative state the substituted judgement test is the correct test to apply. The problems with applying a hybrid test to such cases were summed up in the later New Jersey Supreme Court decision in *In Re Jobes*:

'While a benefits-burden analysis is difficult with marginally competent patients … it is essentially impossible with patients in a persistent vegetative state. By definition, such patients … do not experience any of the benefits or burdens that the Conroy balancing tests are intended or able to appraise. Therefore, we hold that these tests should not be applied to patients in the persistent vegetative state.' (529 A. 2d, p. 419 [1987])

A fortiori, this applies to the application of the common law best interests test to the patient in a persistent vegetative state. At that point the patient arguably has no interests to be maintained and as such the test becomes redundant. The very fact that courts persist in using such outmoded tools in this area of decision-making demonstrates the limits of the judicial role in the absence of more sophisticated statutorily defined tests. It is akin to using a knife to conduct a delicate piece of surgery where laser equipment is more appropriate. These tests, developed in an age where the interests of the individual were far from paramount, gave the impression of justice where in fact what was being decided was the redistribution of an incompetent person's wealth. Similarly, today we use the term 'best interests' to cover a multitude of gaps in the creaking machinery of the common law. Harmon has expressed eloquently the difficulties in applying extant common law tests to the patient in a persistent vegetative state:

'Common law would not have a name for [the PVS patient]. Certainly, she was not an idiot. While her condition was now static, she had not come into the world with a deficient mental apparatus ... neither was she a lunatic. Although she had once been competent, there was no waxing and waning of her intellect. Indeed, there was no longer any intellect at all. [Her] deficit was more profound than the lunatic's was. His was a failure of reason alone; hers was a failure of consciousness ... the persistence of her lower brain function and the presence of her warm body made her not dead, not alive, not an idiot, not a lunatic. There was a lacuna in the language of the law, so she was thrown into the general class of incompetents. There was no fine-tuning as to who was in that class – just individuals who were presently incompetent, regardless of how they came to be that way.' (Harmon, 'Falling off the Vine: Legal Fictions and the Doctrine of Substituted Judgement', *Yale Law Journal*, pp. 37-8)

In Ireland, the courts were also forced to use the extant common law machinery in developing a test in this area. In the

Supreme Court, the order of Justice Lynch in the High Court was upheld, but the court applied a discrete 'best interests' test rather than the hybrid model favoured by Justice Lynch. It could be suggested that at first sight, the common law 'best interests' standard may be rather objective in nature, in that it does not focus on how the patient would have chosen, if the patient was capable of so doing, but rather on the decision which is most in keeping with the welfare of the patient. However, it has been argued that this standard strays too far away from the ideal of patient autonomy and that indeed one may be confusing other interests with the 'best interests' of the patient. The major problem with the 'best interests' test is that the 'best interests' as identified by the court may not necessarily coincide with the individual patient's interests but rather the 'best interests' of the patient as perceived by third parties such as the medical profession and the judiciary. As Minow has observed:

'To speak of "best interests" also veils the very present risk that the decision will fall short of its name. For this reason, some scholars have advocated replacing the term … with the phrase "least detrimental alternative". This phrase may at least humble the decision-maker with the recognition that any [patient] in need of such a determination is already far from his or her best interests.' (Minow, *Making All the Difference*, p. 325)

The judicial track record in this area tends to certain disequilibrium in favour of professionally perceived best interests rather than the individual patient's best interests. Thus, as Teff has noted:

'Treatment in the "best interests" of the patient sounds like a very reassuring criterion; deceptively so, when one appreciates that it can be satisfied by a medical judgement which the court and even the preponderance of expert medical opinion would have rejected.' (Teff, *Reasonable Care*, p. 41)

The fact that the court acknowledges that it is in the best interest to die in such cases is not necessarily determinative of a happy ending to the story. The reality of death from treatment withdrawal falls more readily into Minow's notion of the 'least detrimental alternative' or as Margaret Pabst Battin's terms it the 'least worst death' (Pabst Battin, *The Least Worst Death*, p. 34). Thus, according to Battin:

> 'Because the laws actually protect only refusal of treatment, they can hardly guarantee a peaceful, easy death. Thus, we see a widening gulf between the intent of the law to protect the patient's final desires and the outcomes if the law is actually followed. The physician is caught in between: he or she recognises the patient's right to die peacefully, naturally, and with whatever dignity is possible, but foresees the unfortunate results that may come about when the patient exercises this right as the law permits.' (Pabst Battin, *The Least Worst Death*, p. 35)

The reality of death by treatment withdrawal is therefore masked by legal rhetoric.

Doctors Differ, Patients do not Die: Rights, Resistance and Counter-Hegemony

The further reification of the patient in this case occurred in the aftermath of the Supreme Court's decision. The pro-life lobby reacted by stating that this was unacceptable erosion of the principle of the sanctity of life. The reaction of many healthcare professionals was antipathetic to the judgement (Costello, 'Supreme Court decision "a clear case of euthanasia"', *The Cork Examiner*, 28 July 1995, p. 4). Indeed, in statements issued in the wake of the Supreme Court's decision in *Re A Ward of Court*, both the Irish Medical Council and the Irish Nursing Board were of the view that it is not ethical for a doctor or a nurse to withdraw artificial hydration or nutrition from a patient who is not dying. (Irish Medical Council, *Statement of the Council after their Statutory Meeting on 4th April, 1995*; Irish Nursing Board, *Guidance of the Irish Nursing Board of 18th August, 1995*) It would appear that the Irish Medical Council seems to disregard the approach taken by the Supreme Court in relation to treatment withdrawal by announcing that:

'It is the view of the Council that access to nutrition and hydration is one of the basic needs of human beings. This remains so even when, from time to time, this need can only be fulfilled by means of long established methods such as nasogastric and gastronomy tube feeding.' (Irish Medical Council, *Statement of the Council after their Statutory Meeting on 4th April, 1995*)

In the statement issued by the Medical Council in response to the Supreme Court's decision on treatment withdrawal, the Council, by quoting selectively from its *Guide to Ethical Conduct and Behaviour and to Fitness to Practise* criticised implicitly the stance taken by the Supreme Court. Thus, the inclusion in the statement of the following paragraph from the ethical guidelines can only be seen as a veiled attack on the Supreme Court's decision: 'Medical care must not be used as a tool of the State to be granted or withheld or altered in character under political pressure.' (Irish Medical Council, *A Guide to Ethical Conduct and Behaviour and to Fitness to Practise*, par. 12. 05)

Similarly in its latest set of ethical guidelines the Medical Council notes in paragraph 24. 1 under the heading of Inability to Communicate and Consent states:

'For the seriously ill patient who is unable to communicate or understand, it is desirable that the doctor discusses management with the next of kin or the legal guardians prior to reaching a decision about the use or non-use of treatments *which will not contribute to recovery from the primary illness*. The Council reiterates its view that access to nutrition and hydration remain one of the basic needs of human needs, and all reasonable and practical efforts should be made to maintain both of them.' (Irish Medical Council, *A Guide to Ethical Conduct and Behaviour and to Fitness to Practise*, p. 38)

This guideline appears to be widely drawn enough in the first sentence to allow for the respecting of a patient's previously made decisions about healthcare, yet in the second sentence the Council adds a rather dogmatic statement about the need to maintain water and nutrition which is a direct reference to its

1995 reaction to the ward case which would appear to militate against an individual's previously expressed wishes to be respected. Moreover, this mere statement of principle falls far short of the detailed practical guidance required in such cases. Rather than engaging in a game of bush warfare with the legal and policy actors, the medical profession should be engaging in constructive dialogue with legal professionals and policy-makers in an attempt to create some workable framework in relation to patient decision-making in the area of treatment withdrawal and treatment withholding. Professional organisations in other jurisdictions have recognised the need for detailed and constructive debate in this area of medical practice and have not attempted to bury the issue in gnomic references to ethical propriety. Such signalling of ethical disapproval is not acceptable when faced with the complex issues of fact and law raised by this aspect of medical treatment. The reference in the guidelines to the importance of access to artificial nutrition and hydration seems to contradict the previous statement which refers to treatments which will not contribute to recovery from the primary illness. Surely artificial hydration and nutrition do not contribute to recovery from brain injury, but rather merely prolong the patient's suspension in a persistent vegetative state. It leads one to conclude that the Council is drawing a sharp distinction between treatment on the one hand and artificial nutrition and hydration on the other. This, with respect, is again not a constructive contribution to the resolution of such ethical dilemmas. This bears out a certain dichotomous attitude on the part of medical professionals to artificial hydration on the one hand, and what are regarded as more invasive treatments like dialysis and ventilation on the other. In the United States, a number of empirical studies found that doctors who treat children are reluctant to discontinue medically provided nutrition, yet at the same time are willing to forego other forms of life-sustaining treatment such as ventilators or cardiopulmonary resuscitation. This is attributed to an emotional reaction which the authors of the studies claim has acquired undeserved ethical plausibility. The authors argue that the critical moral question is not how simple, how natural, how customary, how invasive, how expensive a treatment may be, but rather whether the treatment – whatever its characteristics – is likely to provide the patient with benefits that are sufficient to make it worthwhile to endure the burdens that accompany such intervention. (British Medical Association, *Withdrawing and Withholding Treatment: A Consultation Paper from the BMA's Medical Ethics Committee*)

This negative reaction to the right to treatment withdrawal was similar to the Medical Council's reaction to the Supreme Court's decision in *Attorney-General v X.* ([1992] 1 IR.1) In the aftermath of that decision, the Medical Council took an equally divergent stance by announcing that doctors who performed abortions were acting unethically (Irish Medical Council, *A Guide to Ethical Conduct and Behaviour*, p. 36). This policy is maintained in the latest set of ethical guidelines. On the level of legal discourse as reflected in cases like *Re A Ward of Court,* the emphasis is on the idea of patient autonomy. However, at the level of professional discourse, the emphasis continues to be placed on beneficence rather than patient autonomy. The patient who desires to cease artificial hydration or nutrition continues to have his wishes ignored in the traditionalist discourse of the medical and nursing professions. Indeed the medical and nursing professions resisted the Supreme Court's decision to such an extent that the ward died at home in the care of her relatives as no hospital would carry out the court order to withdraw treatment. This reflects Bataille's scenario wherein 'The idea of a world where human life might be artificially prolonged has a nightmare quality' (Bataille, *Eroticism,* p. 101). Even more nightmarish is a world where conflicting elite constructions of the valid death ignore the individual patient.

Thus, in reality the ability to exercise autonomy in relation to the right to die in the healthcare context is constrained first and foremost by the healthcare professions' conception of morality rather than by Roman Catholic dogma *per se*. This is not to say that the Roman Catholic Church does not maintain a certain influence in this area. However, today, it may be more correct to state that the notions of morality held by professional groups and lay pro-life groups have filled the vacuum left in public discourse by the diminishing role played by the institutional church in the formulation of public policy on areas of moral controversy. The Supreme Court's activist stance has resulted in an apparent shift on the symbolic level to a less conservative model of the right to life, but has led to little change in terms of being actually able to exercise one's right to die due to the barriers erected by the antithetical views of certain groups in society. This can be seen from the evidence of theologians in the ward case. The debate even in theological circles as to what theology allowed in this area was far from uniform.

The residual importance of the influence of the Roman Catholic Church on issues of moral controversy can be witnessed by the fact that in the High Court hearing of *Re A Ward of Court*, moral theologians from the Roman Catholic Church were called to give evidence in relation to the morality of treatment withdrawal. In addition, Justice Lynch received a working paper from the Church of Ireland detailing its view on euthanasia. Justice Lynch gave the following justification for allowing the hearing of evidence in relation to the ethics of euthanasia:

'The evidence of the moral theologians is of relevance for two reasons: first, as showing that in proposing the course which they do propose the Ward's family are not contravening their own ethic ... and secondly, the matter being res integra, the views of theologians of various faiths are of assistance in that they endeavour to apply right reason to the problems for decision by the Court and analogous problems.' ([1995 2 ILRM 401, p. 453-4)

Two Roman Catholic theologians were called to give evidence on behalf of the ward's family. They were both of the view that the family's desire to have treatment withdrawn was in keeping with Roman Catholic moral guidance on the issue. However, another Roman Catholic theologian who gave evidence on behalf of the institution in which the ward was being treated argued that this was not the case. This demonstrates that while there may be division within the Roman Catholic Church on the issue, the eventual decision arrived at by both the High Court and the Supreme Court in this case is not antithetical to Roman Catholic moral teaching. However, those like pro-life groups and healthcare professionals who have not been acculturated into the intricacies of Roman Catholic theology have argued that such an outcome is antithetical to traditional cultural values as opposed to religious values *per se*. This is not a rigorous philosophical or theological stance, but one based on a perceived notion of traditional Irish societal values and further complicates the Irish debate on death and dying.

This reflects the reality that we are not appealing to some immutable moral good but rather to the definition of an immutable moral good applied by those who hold power at any given moment. Thus, the [Roman Catholic] Church applied an interpretation of the good that excluded such intervention, as did the healthcare professions. This was opposed to the Supreme Court's reasoning, which spoke of an individual rights based notion of the good. What is most troubling is the fact that those who objected to the legal decision were those who had the power of translating the abstract right into reality, the medical and nursing professions. Without some form of co-operation from the professions, the likelihood of such rights being secured in reality were slim. This created a resistance to the legal discourse of individual rights in favour of a more communitarian model of the common good, which was informed by an appeal to traditional ethical values. O'Mahony and Delanty have noted this cultural schizophrenia in Ireland, the bizarre mingling of the modern and the pre-modern:

'A society began to take shape that could live with the most glaring contradictions. The development path of post-war Ireland began in the late 1940s to create the central contradiction of the last forty or so years of the century. It firstly took the form of hesitant enclaves of modern values within the traditional, anti-modern order and it later began to take its

present form with modern values in the ascendant but compromised by the power of tradition.' (O'Mahony and Delanty,
Rethinking Irish History, p. 167)

Being compromised by the power of tradition is the common
theme in the area of bioethics debates in Ireland. In all areas of
medical treatment, individual choice is constantly disrupted by
the power of tradition, even when this tradition has been quest-
ioned and found wanting by many in society and has even been
rejected by the courts.

Treatment Withdrawal, Where Next? Legislative and Institutional Options

While cases like *Re A Ward of Court* have been important in developing an Irish medical jurisprudence, they must only be regarded as tentative first steps in the direction of a comprehensive response to the many questions which this area of medical
treatment raises. Indeed, in *Re A Ward of Court* it was pointed out
in the Supreme Court decision by Justice O'Flaherty that the
case was not to be viewed as a general precedent:

'It is of the utmost importance to state that we are deciding
this case on a specific set of facts. It must be clear that our decision should not be regarded as authority for anything
wider than the case with which we are confronted.' (1995 2
ILRM 401, p. 431, see also the judgements of Chief Justice
Hamilton at p. 423 and Justice Blayney at p. 444)

These statements may in and of themselves be seen as the
best argument for the introduction of a more detailed statutory
framework in this area. By stating this the court is admitting the
limits of the piecemeal approach of the common law. Thus,
while in common law and in constitutional law the broad principle of a right to refuse medical treatment, where the patient's
best interests warrant it, has been recognised, outstanding questions remain which can only be answered by more specific legislative and ethical guidance. Thus, what types of cases, other
than the near PVS patient, fall into the category of patients protected by this right? What about cases of stroke victims and

those suffering from profound dementia who display multiple morbidity? What do best interests really mean in such a case and how should they be applied? Are there any detailed professional guidelines in this area, which would aid the courts in the decision-making process?

The British Medical Association has provided a helpful advice in relation to the problem of which conditions should be included within the scope of such decisions. They state that it is not the label attached to the condition which should determine whether non-treatment was justified but rather such decisions should be based on the demonstrable irreversibility of damage to specific neural pathways (British Medical Association, *Withdrawing and Withholding Treatment*). This approach provides much more constructive guidance than merely stating that everything should be solved on a case by case basis. In addition, the question of whether the principle of the right to withdraw treatment should apply to cases of treatment withholding or selective non-treatment may also arise. Again, the general principle of weighing up whether treatment should be given in the patient's best interests could be applied to this area. Obviously rather than wait for a specific case to come before the courts for decision, legislation and detailed professional guidelines would be a preferable option.

In the 1996 English decision in the case of *Re R (Adult: Medical Treatment)* ([1996] 2 FLR 99) some guidance was given as to how to proceed in such cases. R was a twenty-three-year-old male born with severe brain malformation and cerebral palsy. In addition he suffered from epilepsy, was blind, deaf, incontinent and was unable to walk or sit upright unaided. He was unable to communicate or to have any consistent interactions with his social environment. He was not in a persistent vegetative state but was described as being in a state of low awareness and operated cognitively and neurologically at the level of a newborn infant. His GP believed that his condition was deteriorating both physically and neurologically as he suffered from recurrent chest infections, which required repeated admission to hospital.

At the time of the case he weighed only five stone and suffered from dehydration. His hospital consultant told the court that it would be unethical to continue to treat R actively and that it was in his best interests to allow nature to take its course the next time R had a life-threatening crisis. Both R's family and the rest of the healthcare team were in agreement with this prognosis. However, the Disability Law Agency took the case to court stating that it was in his best interests to continue the treatment. The court held that it was lawful and in R's best interests for cardiopulmonary resuscitation to be withheld and for antibiotics to be withheld if R were to develop a potentially life threatening infection. The court, in distinguishing artificial hydration and nutrition as falling into a different category, authorised a gastronomy tube to be inserted in R.

In reaching this decision, the court was able to rely on the 1993 guidelines of the BMA and the Royal College of Nursing on Cardiopulmonary Resuscitation (British Medical Association and Royal College of Nursing, *Decisions Relating to Cardiopulmonary Resuscitation: A Statement from the BMA and the RCN in association with the Resuscitation Council*). These guidelines, while dealing specifically with CPR, can be adapted to a variety of other life-sustaining procedures and could be used as a basis for decision-making in this area:

1. Non-treatment decisions should be considered where:

(a) A patient's condition indicates that treatment is unlikely to be successful;

(b) The treatment is contrary to the patient's previously expressed wish;

(c) The treatment is likely to be followed by a quality of life, which would not be acceptable to the patient.

2. There is a presumption in favour of life-sustaining treatment in emergency situations where no prior decision has been made about the appropriateness of the treatment and the patient's wishes are unknown.

3. Responsibility for a treatment decision rests with the clinician in charge of the patient's care. The decision should only

be made after wide consultation and consideration of all aspects of the patient's condition. The clinician in charge must be prepared to discuss the decision with other health professionals involved with the patient. The patient's known views and the views of the patient's friends and relatives must also be taken into account.

4. When the non-treatment decision is based on a clinical judgement that there is unlikely to be any medical benefit from the treatment, there must, wherever possible, be discussions with the patient, or with people close to the patient, to try and ensure that they understand why such treatment would be clinically inappropriate.

5. If the non-treatment decision is based on quality of life considerations, the views of the patient where they can be ascertained are particularly important. If the patient's views cannot be discovered, the opinion of people close to the patient may be helpful in determining the patient's best interests. (British Medical Association and Royal College of Nursing, *Decisions Relating to Cardiopulmonary Resuscitation: A Statement from the BMA and the RCN in association with the Resuscitation Council*)

This case was an example where legal and medical principles could work together to produce a workable solution to an area of bioethical controversy, rather than acting in an antagonistic manner leading to stasis.

It is clear therefore that the only satisfactory means of dealing with the lacunae which persist in this area is the introduction of legislation. Lord Browne-Wilkinson in his judgement in *Airedale NHS Trust v Bland* offered a convincing argument for a legislative solution to this dilemma:

'It seems to me imperative that the moral, social and legal issues raised by this case should be considered by Parliament ... If Parliament fails to act, then judge-made law will of necessity through a gradual and uncertain process provide a legal answer to each new question as it arises. But in my judgement that is not the best way to proceed ... It is for

Parliament to address the wider problems, which the case raises and lay down principles of law generally applicable to the withdrawal of life support systems.' ([1993] 2 WLR 316, p. 382)

In Ireland, the current state of the law in the area is not satisfactory. A logical and reasonable reaction to the decision in *Re A Ward of Court* would be to enshrine in legislation the right of the individual to make anticipatory decisions about treatment withdrawal. The Supreme Court, as with so many other issues of a medico-ethical nature in Ireland, has been forced to adjudicate due to the failure of legislators to introduce legislation in this field, due to the fear of attracting controversy and losing votes. This failure on the part of the legislature places the judiciary in the invidious position of having to deliberate and reach solutions to highly charged moral as well as legal dilemmas.

Rather than depend on a case by case resolution of the dilemmas posed by treatment withdrawal, the Government could decide to take some responsibility in this field and introduce a programme of legislation which would put the concept of treatment withdrawal on a statutory footing. The first step would be to introduce legislation which would allow for the making of advance directives. This would allow those who are now competent to create a testamentary document which would set out their wishes in relation to medical treatment should they ever enter a state of incapacity.

The principal problem with this method is that those who now lack legal capacity, such as the mentally incompetent and minors, will be unable to avail of this instrument. However, given legal conceptions of rationality and competence this problem is likely to remain. On the positive side, such an initiative would at last give legal recognition to individual autonomy in this area of medical treatment, thus bringing it into line with the consent model as it is understood in the case of the conscious adult and medical treatment. This, it could be argued, is merely an extension of the general right to refuse medical treatment to the area of treatment at the end of life. The patient's wishes could still be ascertained through the medium of the advance directive.

The English Law Commission has proposed a number of key legislative initiatives on the question of anticipatory decision-making in its 1995 *Report on Mental Incapacity*, which have been incorporated in the Government's 1997 green paper on decision-making for the incompetent (Lord Chancellor's Department, *Who Decides?*). The Law Commission recommended that the law in relation to advance directives be put on a statutory footing. It is submitted that the Irish legislature should take a similar approach to the one outlined by the Law Commission in this area of medical practice. As our legislative canon is quite heavily influenced by English legislative conventions, this would not be a radical departure in procedural terms. The recommendations are based on a similar common law tradition and such legislation would not prove difficult to weave into our current statutory framework. What could prove to be a difficulty would be the traditional Irish antipathy to pioneering social legislation that aims to afford greater protection to individual autonomy. One need only look to the current stalemate over proposed legislation in another field of medical controversy – pregnancy termination to satisfy oneself that this would indeed be the case.

A legislative basis for advance refusals of care would give rise to more certainty. The existence of legislation would bolster the common law right to refuse treatment and allow for more detailed guidelines on the issue. The principle that the Law Commission sought to uphold in recommending such a move was that patients should be enabled and encouraged to exercise genuine choice about treatments and procedures. The introduction of legislation in this area, while clarifying the present position, may also be subject to the extant problem where the refusal of treatment may conflict with the views of the medical professionals caring for the patient. In this regard, an advance directive would not require a doctor to act unlawfully or force a doctor to provide treatment that is not in the patient's best interests. Moreover, as the Commission's proposals envisioned that the healthcare professional would act in the best interests of the patient in interpreting any advance statements made by the patient when she was competent so to do. The Law Commission included within the scope of best interests, the patient's past and present wishes, feelings and the factors which she would consider, the need to permit and encourage patients to participate in treatment decisions, the views of other appropriate people and the availability of an effective less restrictive option. This statutory best interests test would thus address the actual situation in which the patient found herself and allows the decision to be made in the current context rather than in a vacuum. Moreover, it would allow those charged with the patient's care to address issue of new treatments, which had been developed since the patient made the advance statement. Thus, as the UK Government Green Paper points out, a doctor would be under an obligation to consider whether the new treatment is something the patient would have wished to consider had they known about it (Lord Chancellor's Department, *Who Decides?* par. 4. 17). Appropriate people to consult in such a situation would be family members or other carers. Thus as the Green Paper notes, the decision is not to be seen in isolation 'but against a background of doctor/patient dialogue' (Lord Chancellor's Department, *Who Decides?* par. 4. 18). The introduction of legislation on advance directives will not rule out court involvement entirely. It will still be necessary in cases of doubt or ambiguity in relation to the advance directive, or in cases where there was a question as to whether or not it had been withdrawn.

In addition, it is submitted that the Irish Medical Council should take note of the recent initiative undertaken by the British Medical Association in producing a Code of Practice in relation to advance statements about healthcare, and perhaps establish a steering group on the lines of the British Medical Association to study the issue and to produce professional guidelines on advance directives (British Medical Association, *Advance Statements about Medical Treatment: Code of Practice*). This on its own is of little value, however, if parliament does not act by introducing legislation that would clarify the legal position of the advance directive.

A complementary form of legislation, which could also be introduced, is the idea of a healthcare enduring power of attorney. In Ireland, the law in relation to powers of attorney is contained in the Powers of Attorney Act 1996. This Act provides, *inter alia*, for the creation of an enduring power of attorney. This form of power of attorney allows the power to endure after the donor of the power has become mentally incapacitated. However, the enduring power of attorney extends only to property, business or financial affairs and personal care decisions. Section 4 of the Act defines personal care decisions as follows:

(a) Where the donor should live;

(b) With whom the donor should live;

(c) Whom the donor should see and not see;

(d) What training or rehabilitation the donor should get;

(e) The donor's diet and dress;

(f) Inspection of the donor's personal papers;

(g) Housing, social welfare and other benefits for the donor;

Decisions in relation to healthcare or medical treatment are not included within the ambit of the enduring power of attorney as currently understood.

The principal obstacle to the legal recognition of a healthcare power of attorney in the case of a patient who, for example, enters a permanent state of unconsciousness or the introduction of living will legislation would appear to be government's reluctance to recognise that a detailed statutory framework is required to deal with the complex issues of fact and law that may arise in this area of medical treatment.

Conclusion

Like Fintan O'Toole's conclusion in relation to the current state of Irish society, we are also at a key moment in the evolution of bioethics in Irish society. Depending on the route we take, we can either create a climate where individual choice is respected in the area of medical treatment or where patient choice is subordinated to other interests. This can be achieved through wide-ranging debate on the issues, including consultation with the public, policymakers, healthcare professionals, and legal professionals, in order to come to a reasoned compromise which takes into account the reality of the choices faced by patients in this area and the responsibilities of the professionals who are charged with their care. In other words, bioethics should be taken seriously rather than as a forum for political and moral conflict, which finally produces no resolution of the dilemmas, faced daily by patients and healthcare professionals. Alternatively, we can engage in 'the Irish solution to an Irish problem' attitude which we have excelled in the last thirty years – either ignoring the issue or deftly sidestepping it in legislation, which aimed at pleasing all but in the end proved ineffectual. A case in point is The Abortion Information Act with its jesuitical distinction between abortion referral and information, allowing the latter but preventing the former. Another case of one step forward and two steps back. This approach is not confronting an issue and attempting to bring about a resolution, it is merely legislative abdication. Moreover, strategies by some groups in society of demonising those who attempt to provide a pragmatic and democratic framework for the resolution of such bioethical dilemmas is self-defeating. It leads to a society engaged in a perpetual conflict over rigid values and to the politics of symbolic posturing. We have seen in Northern Ireland the human cost of this politics of intractability. There must be a third way, a means of focusing one's energies on a common solution to such deep-seated conflict.

There is a choice to be made as to the model which will form the basis for legal intervention in the area of death and dying in Ireland. On the one hand, one can choose the model of the natural death. This model is rooted in deontological ideas about the intrinsic value of life as an abstract ideal. The natural death model is the offspring of the sanctity of life model and is thus absolutist and impersonal. The sanctity of life model has been the dominant model in Irish legal discourse on the topic of the right to life to date. This model, rather than being a flexible one adapting to the needs of an evolving societal framework, is absolutist. In other words, it fits into Ronald Dworkin's model of the 'constitution of detail' (Dworkin, *Life's Dominion*, p.119). This model is hardly the model which would fit very easily into the medical law context. Medical law is concerned with often quite complex fact situations involving, *inter alia*, important questions of personal autonomy. As a result, the wishes and desires of the individual patient must be taken into account, not in a perfunctory manner, but in a manner which best serves the autonomy of the patient, while not forgetting the interests of the healthcare provider. Applying a deontological model to this scenario may serve the purpose of upholding the ideal of the sanctity of life, but it does not uphold the equally important ideal of patient autonomy.

That this model poorly serves individual autonomy can be seen in the manner in which both the courts and the legislature have dealt with issues in the sphere of medical practice. Thus the issue of abortion clearly demonstrated the important practical ramifications of applying a deontological model to a question of individual autonomy. The patient and doctor, the central participants in this therapeutic relationship have, within this model, been relegated to the status of mere bit-players, performing roles which are neither respectful of individual autonomy nor the dignity of the person.

In recent years, this deontological model has been subject to challenge from another model, which appears to offer more in terms of respecting individual autonomy. Thus, having witnessed the case of *Attorney-General v X and Others* and that of *Re A Ward of Court*, one could argue that Irish law, in the zone of individual rights, may be commencing to question the previous paradigm of the sanctity of life in more vehement terms than heretofore.

Like Irish society, Irish law in this zone, it could be argued, is undergoing a difficult metamorphosis from the paradigm of the natural to that of the post-natural or, as the French philosopher

Gilles Lipovetsky has termed it, a post-moralistic state (Lipovetsky, 1991, p. 176). What the post-natural phase of Irish individual rights jurisprudence holds will be dependent on individuals rather than on the moral collectivity. It is to be hoped that the transition will lead to a new autonomy, this time personal rather than political.

That it is important to identify a model, which will underpin any future Irish jurisprudence on death, is clear. The phenomenon of the legal appropriation of death is a societal reality from which Ireland is not immune. In the face of the very real policy and personal ramifications of the issues which arise from this phenomenon, how have legal and policy actors in Ireland reacted? It has to be said not very well. The country has, in effect, no policy framework within which to resolve the complex dilemmas in this area of medical practice.

The Supreme Court's decision in *Re A Ward of Court* has accelerated the need for a legislative response to the question of treatment withdrawal, by putting in place legislation in the area of advance directives which would give legal reality to the ideal of individual autonomy at life's end. Detailed legislative guidance on the issue is crucial, both for the patient and for the healthcare professional who is daily faced with such dilemmas.

CHAPTER EIGHT

Genetics and the Future of the Person

Sheila Greene

In 1999 genetics and genetic engineering are certainly very much in the news. A very heated debate, which involves many sections of the community – farmers, big business, politicians, scientists and consumers – is ongoing in relation to genetically modified food. People also have become more aware of the advances in genetics that involve manipulation of animal and human genes, particularly highlighted by the birth of Dolly, the cloned sheep, which was announced in February 1997 (Wilmut et al., *Nature*, pp. 810-13). As we await the end of the twentieth century and the beginning of the twenty-first century, there is understandable concern about what this new knowledge and its associated new technologies will bring – will it be good for humanity, will it be bad? Will there be fundamental changes to our way of life and to what it means to be human?

In this paper I wish to explore the nature of the challenge that advances in genetics present to us. I cannot begin to answer questions about whether these advances are for good or for ill, but I will argue that we are on the brink of barely imaginable possibilities in terms of the manipulation of human life. How we use the knowledge and technology, which are capable of transforming the possibilities into realities, is, or should be, the responsibility of us all.

In the wealthy parts of this world we are living in a time of extraordinarily rapid change. Fifty years ago it would have been unimaginable to all but the futurists and the writers of science fiction that ordinary people would have computers in their homes capable of holding and processing more information than the then existing computers which occupied an entire floor of a building. Computers of today are one hundred million times more powerful for the same unit cost than they were fifty years ago. In 1990, communication by mobile phones and email was a novelty, but it is now commonplace. The World Wide Web was not introduced until 1994; now even primary schools have their own web pages. The nature of work and the nature of communication have changed in a very short time beyond recognition and these changes also influence how we behave and how we see others and ourselves. Any vision of the future needs to take account of the revolution in computational technology even where the focus of discussion is biotechnology, since the two will in the foreseeable future work hand in hand. In the long run, it is hard to know whether the transformation of humans will be by means of electronic implants and extensions or by the products of biological and genetic engineering or a combination of both.

With reference to the future of computational science, the computer inventor Ray Kurtzweil states, 'the primary political and philosophical issue of the next century will be the definition of who we are.' (Kurweil, *The Age of Spiritual Machines*, p. 2) He believes that by 2030 we will have invented self-conscious machines and electronic extensions and enhancements of our own bodies that will cause us to question the definition of personhood. Alongside these developments in computer technology we have the developments in biotechnology, which are the focus of this paper. We are on the brink of a future where our ideas about humanity and personhood are about to be challenged as never before because of the sophistication and precision of these new technologies.

Using our ingenuity and inventiveness to change and enhance our bodies, to improve on nature, is certainly not new. As a species it is part of what defines us. Our intelligence allows us to adapt to our environment and also to invent. For tens of thousands of years we have re-shaped our environment and re-shaped ourselves; we aren't about to stop now.

In order to predict how we will handle the new technologies

and the discoveries of genetics it is important to place these discoveries in their social context and to take into account the kind
of society and mores which prevail in late twentieth century
capitalist democracies. It has been argued that one of the major
consequences of the combined impact of the communications
revolution and the consumer society is that we are so over-
whelmed by choice and possibility, that in relation to our sense of
who we are we no longer have a sense of self as fixed and stable.
In a way that our ancestors could not, we can play with our own
idea of self. We can, in the middle of a city like Dublin, eat Thai
food, watch Italian movies, decorate our homes according to the
principles of feng shui and dress like American baseball players.
We can invent and reinvent ourselves according to images presented on television or the Internet or concocted by our well-fed
imaginations. We can make choices that were not possible before, such as the choice to be sexually active but not to become a
parent, the choice to fight signs of ageing by paying for cosmetic
surgery. Of course there are huge constraints: some people are
too poor to avail of all that is on offer. And what is on offer is itself restricted to what our consumer society makes available to
us: thus we may have a choice between twenty different colours
of bathroom towel but no choice between chemically contami-
nated and pure water. But we are getting used to the benefits
and excitements of technological advance and we are getting
used to the kind of choices it can offer us.

We are also getting used to the idea that science and medical
science will give us control over those aspects of nature that can
cause us distress. For example, we are already used to the idea of
reproductive technologies which allow us to circumvent problems which would once have prevented men and women from
becoming parents. And now it looks as though science may offer
us conquest over those aspects of life which were previously un-
controllable – inherited illnesses and disabilities, cancer, ageing
and even death itself.

It is in this context that we must place discussion about the
impact of recent advances in genetics. We expect science to keep

on advancing and we expect to reap the benefits of that advance. We expect to be able to exercise our rights and our preferences. At the same time we are wary and remember the times when the scientists were full of reassurances but the consequences of their discoveries and their interventions were disastrous, as with Thalidomide or BSE.

I will now look at some of the recent developments in genetics that will make our capacity to interfere with nature even more precise and sophisticated than before. Some of these developments are placed under the heading of the new genetics. New genetics is the recent developments in molecular genetics – dating from the discovery of the molecular structure of DNA in 1953 – which permit identification of individual genes and which in certain circumstances will permit the selection and elimination of genes or the recombining of genes, the kind of genetic engineering we see already in plants. Cloning is, of course, another remarkable advance but it does not come under the heading of molecular genetics. It depends on a knowledge of genetics but is another example of the kind of reproductive technologies which have been with us for years, starting with the identification of chromosomal abnormalities like Down's Syndrome and moving on to interventions aimed at addressing infertility such as Artificial Insemination by Donor and In-Vitro Fertilisation.

Cloning involves the taking of a cell, any kind of cell other than a germ cell, from a mature organism, let us say a sheep, and placing the cell nucleus which contains the DNA of that animal into an egg of another animal which has been emptied of its nucleus. The egg will sometimes start to develop in the same way as a normally fertilised egg develops. The technology is far from perfect. To produce Dolly took 277 fusions between eggs and cells. Only twenty-nine started to develop and became embryos that were implanted into thirteen different ewes. One ewe became pregnant and produced Dolly. However, despite the apparent imperfection of the technology to date, the knowledge exists which will enable some scientist somewhere to produce the first cloned baby. As far as we know it has not happened yet. The USA and most European states have agreed to a moratorium on human cloning. For most doctors and scientists who might have the skills and knowledge to engage in such research, the whole area is out of bounds.

Judging by the public reaction to the news of Dolly's birth and the evident implication that human cloning was now around the corner, it seemed that many people found the idea of human cloning frightening or repellent or both. However, a recent survey showed that seven per cent of a representative sample of US citizens found human cloning thoroughly acceptable. The famous sociobiologist Richard Dawkins has recently stated that he would find the idea of cloning his own daughter acceptable in some circumstances. And what are these circumstances and how soon will people be demanding, expecting access to this technology? And for how long will unscrupulous doctors hold out against the temptations of the great financial rewards that will be made available to them? Within two weeks of the announcement of Dolly's arrival a company called Clonaid based in the Bahamas was offering its services on the Internet. For a fee of $200,000 they advertised a fantastic opportunity to parents with fertility problems or homosexual couples to have a child cloned from one of them (Silver, *Remaking Eden,* p. 123). In South Korea in 1998, a cloned human embryo from the somatic cell of a thirty-year-old woman was developed up to the four-cell stage and then destroyed. In the USA, Dr Richard Seed has announced his intention of cloning babies for infertile couples and his intention of getting round the USA's five-year moratorium by moving to Japan.

Despite a continuing repugnance in some government and scientific circles to the idea of reproductive cloning, there seems to be a more widespread acceptance of the cloning of stem cells to produce spare parts. In the UK the Cloning Working Group of the Human Genetics Advisory Commission has recommended a ban on reproductive cloning but also recommends that cloning research using human embryos should be permitted. This research involves the cloning of embryo cells that could be used to produce duplicate organs, skin and other tissues.

In relation to reproductive cloning, many of the concerns expressed centred around the idea of clones as replica persons, exact copies of the original in every respect. Is a clone a total replica of its parent? Genetically it is a replica, but of course it will not be in any way the same person as its parent, no more than two identical twins are the same person. In fact the similarity in phenotype will be less, in two main ways. First the cellular context for the cloned nucleus will be different from that which surrounded the original nucleus, and secondly the environment for the cloned baby will be more different than the environment of identical twins reared together. A cloned baby, unaware of his or her status and not subject to different treatment because of his or her cloned status, would therefore live a life no different from any of us and would be very different from the parent in many ways, while sharing some obvious similarities in appearance and other less definitive similarities in temperament and ability. What we care to make of this is the important issue. The discourses that cluster around the field of genetics can promote a view of the person as being entirely determined by his or her genes. I would be concerned that in the present era where we have seen an upsurge in the popularity of biological determinism, genes are given a primacy they do not warrant (Green, 'What Make a Person a Person? The Limits and Limitations of Genetics' in Designing Life?, 1999). Because one faulty gene can have devastating consequences for a person's physical and mental development does not mean that in the normally functioning person genes are the major determining factor in the creation of the adult person and his or her distinctive personality. Indeed they are only part of the story for those who are affected by a damaging gene. Thus the interests, abilities and personalities of children suffering from cystic fibrosis are as various as those of children who have been in car accidents, for example. Identical twins, while looking very similar, often have very different personalities. But as a society we seem increasingly convinced that our genes *are* us. The books of people like Richard Dawkins, promoter of selfish gene theory, become bestsellers (Dawkins, 2nd ed., *The Selfish Gene*). Steven Pinker, evolutionary psychologist and author of *How the Mind Works* is treated like an international superstar. In 1994 an otherwise thoughtful piece by Kathryn Holmquist of *The Irish Times* on the appointment of a clinical geneticist to Our Lady's Hospital in Crumlin, Dublin, was headlined 'Our fate lies in our genes'. Recently I heard a doctor on the radio refer to 'the genetic blueprint which makes us what we are'. We have seen in recent years the resurgence of biological determinism, the view that we are – as Dawkins puts it – nothing but the 'lumbering robot' carriers of our genes (Dawkins, 2nd ed., *The Selfish Gene*, p. 19). Our valuation of ourselves and others as unique and worthy of total respect is fundamentally undermined by such a demeaning and reductive definition of the human. In my opinion, biological determinism is both wrong as an account of what makes us what we are and dangerous.

Biological reductionism disregards the reality that genes are only part of the picture. As the poet, Adrienne Rich comments:

Neither men nor women are merely the enlargement of the contact sheet of genetic encoding, biological givens. Experience shapes us; randomness shapes us, the stars and the weather, our own accommodations and rebellions, above all the social order around us. (Rich, 2nd ed., *Of Woman Born*, p. xv)

In a paper that refers to the future of the person it is necessary to pause and ask what we mean by this term. What is a person? The *Shorter Oxford English Dictionary* defines a person as simply, 'an individual human being; a man, woman or child'.

Philosophers and theologians have spent much time and energy on exploring issues around the definition of personhood. In the library I found two recent books with the same title, *What is a Person?* (Doran, 1989; Goodman, 1988). They and other related texts make fascinating reading. Doran's book starts with the words, 'In the discussion of many contemporary issues, notably in areas such as medical ethics and human rights, a good deal depends on having an accurate and properly defined concept of a person.' (Doran, *What is a Person?*, p. vii) A sensible starting point one might think, but in the margin someone has written, in pencil, 'There is no one definition!' And that is my own conclusion. Broadly I would go along with the *Oxford English Dictionary* – a person is a recognisably human entity. When we start adding attributes such as consciousness, rationality, agency, capacity for reciprocity, the discussion becomes very interesting but the discovery of the essence of personhood retreats further and further into the distance. Some philosophers like Adam Norton claim, 'There is no concept of a person.' (Norton, 'Why There is No Concept of a Person' in *The Person and the Human Mind*) On the other hand, I would think there are myriad concepts of a person. Such concepts vary due to variations in culture and historical period. We construct our notion of personhood. Other cultures and other historical periods have different concepts of the person to those favoured in this era in the West. As the psychologist Bronfenbrenner concludes, 'Human nature, which I had once thought of as a singular noun, turns out to be plural and pluralistic' (Bronfenbrenner, *The Ecology of Human Development*, p. xiii). So it is unlikely that a precise definition can be found which is acceptable universally. Perhaps the best we can do is to adopt a definition which is sufficiently broad to provide us with a starting point for conversation.

There will, for the conceivable future, continue to be entities which are recognisably human and recognisably individual in body and in mind. As Daniel Dennett says, 'At the moment humanity is the deciding mark of personhood' (Dennett, p. 145). Perhaps in the future we will see the development of cyborgs – cybernetic organisms – or intelligent self-conscious machines that demand recognition as human and then may find ourselves asking 'Is this a person?' or 'Is this a human?' Donna Haraway argues that in Western society many of us are living a cyborg existence already – totally engaged with and dependant upon machines of various kinds (Haraway, *Simians, Cyborgs, and Women*). The question has been asked about cloned humans and I think the answer has to be in the affirmative. Cloned human beings, despite being genetic replicas, will be individual human beings since they are recognisably human and are constituted as persons in the same way as all other persons. Solely our genes do not determine our identity as human persons. Solely their genes do not determine the identity as human persons of those who are cloned and there is nothing about the origin or character of their genes which disqualifies them from being human.

The challenge of reproductive cloning is therefore not so much to our definition of personhood but to our valuation of the persons created through cloning. The importance of analysis of what it means to be a person also resides in questions of value and ethics. Thus although definition of the word 'person' may be problematic, issues around how we should behave towards persons or potential persons or rudimentary persons (such as sentient machines?) cannot be avoided and must be debated.

The advent of cloning could possibly raise major issues about the meaning of human life, depending on how we choose to perceive and respond to cloned persons. Cloned babies might be made to feel different by their families or by society. In the science fiction film, *Bladerunner*, cloned humans are called 'replicants', restricted to a four-year life span and treated as slaves. Closer to our present reality, it does not take much imagination to anticipate the possibility that negative reasons for cloning, such as the overwhelming vanity of a parent, might result in the exploitation and instrumentalisation of the cloned child for the parent's ends.

So a cloned human being who is in her form and capacities recognisably human is as much a person as any other. As I see it, there need not be a problem in that cloned being achieving full personhood. Such a problem will only arise *if* society decides that being a clone entails any denial of the normal rights and considerations granted to others. We can decide, as we have decided before, that some people are not persons – they are slaves perhaps, or vermin, or subhuman. In the 1994 Rwandan holocaust the minority Tutsi people were generally referred to as 'cockroaches' by the Hutus (Gourevich, *We Wish To Inform You*

That Tomorrow We Will Be Killed With Our Families: Stories From Rwanda). We are very capable of denying full personhood to others, and cloned humans could join a long list of categories of humans designated by some culture at some time as inferior or unworthy of full human rights and respect.

The other area of extraordinarily rapid advance is at the level of identification of individual genes. The Human Genome Project that will map all 100,000 genes is due to be completed within the next few years. Already genes responsible for a range of disorders have been identified. Clearly if we can identify genes which cause terrible diseases, possibilities open up in terms of intervention to prevent their action. To take the example of Huntington's Disease (HD), it has been known for some time through family studies that this terrible degenerative condition that typically has its onset in adulthood is a hereditary disease that is carried by a dominant gene. This means that if you have the gene you will develop the condition and if one of your parents is affected you have a 50-50 chance of inheriting HD. Much can be done in the way of support for those afflicted by HD and their families but to date all that could be done in terms of prevention was to prevent possible carriers of HD from having children, a very difficult goal to achieve since many possible carriers do not know in their twenties, when they might think about having children, whether they are carriers or not. But now the gene for HD has been found. So was the year 1993 when the gene was identified a time for rejoicing or not? Clearly the discovery of the gene makes it more likely that in future a cure may be found, but for the moment members of families afflicted by HD are faced with terrible dilemmas. If they test prenatally for the presence of a gene and find it means the parent from the HD family is affected, that may be something he or she may or may not want to know. Young adults who face the decision about whether to be tested or not have a hard choice between knowing they will inevitably get HD or knowing they will not, thus putting themselves into a different and perhaps alienated position in relation to the rest of their family. People's reactions to this new genetic information appear to be complex and are only recently being explored by psychologists (e.g. Marteau and Richards, *The Troubled Helix*) but what is very striking, in relation to HD for example, is how few people at risk have taken the test, contrary to the original expectations of some medical practitioners in this area.

The kind of therapeutic interventions which are anticipated for HD will of course be extended to a whole range of other conditions and for any family afflicted with a hereditary condition such advances can only be seen as welcome although, as I have argued, some of the difficulties associated with knowing about your own or your loved one's genetic status are very hard to handle. So there will probably be little disagreement about the desirability of being able to remove or deactivate the gene which causes a disease like HD or Duchenne's Multiple Dystrophy, allowing the treated individual to live a healthy life instead of one blighted and shortened by disease. Where does one draw the line? Many foetuses are aborted each year because they are affected by the chromosomal disorder Down's Syndrome. Yet parents who could not make that choice for lack of information, or chose to continue their pregnancies, will talk about the joy their child has brought them. Others may find the burden of a handicapped child hard to bear, but surely a major part of their problem resides in the lack of support they get from the rest of us? The implication of much of the discussion around medical genetics is that any kind of disability is intolerable and that society cannot but welcome genetic research which eliminates hereditary disability

The negative attitude our society holds towards disability and the disabled are well documented in a paper called 'Abortion and disability: Who should and who should not inhabit the world?' Ruth Hubbard asks, 'Why do we think we have the right to deny life to such people? What does it say to people with disabilities that so much scientific effort is invested in making sure that people like them should never be born? Decisions about what kind of baby to bear are bedevilled by overt and unspoken judgements about which lives are worth living.' (Hubbard, *Abortion and Disability*, p. 199) These are the judgements people make when deciding to terminate a pregnancy and these are the kind of judgements people will make when deciding to make use of the technology of gene therapy.

Although much of the justification for investment in genetic research is couched in terms of its medical benefits, geneticists are not only looking for genes associated with illness. Gene therapy also raises all sorts of possibilities in relation to the obliteration or the enhancement of attributes valued by our society. And for some of the interventions anticipated in the future there will be very few ways in which one could argue that the intervention was medical or therapeutic. Interventions will be conducted in order to subtract a feature seen as socially disadvantageous and/or add a feature that is socially advantageous. Again we see the beginnings of such procedures all round us. Parents want their children to be beautiful and bright. They invest a lot of money and time in straightening their teeth, improving their posture, correcting lisps, and nurturing their intelligence. All very admirable, one might say, as well as a natural desire on the part of parents to give children the best start in life. So, if the technology were to become available would parents choose to eliminate or alter the gene for buckteeth, for shortsightedness? Baldness is hereditary. Will thoughtful parents of the future be expected to ensure the disappearance of the baldness gene? Imagine the irritation of the young man whose parents did not get round to correcting this particular fault. Cher, the pop star and actress who is fifty-two but looks and acts as though she is thirty, is a true twenty-first century woman. She has used her money to replace and enhance her body, removing ribs and flesh, adding silicon. One imagines that she would have little hesitation in availing of the anti-ageing gene, if and when it becomes available, and the hormone therapies and body parts replacement surgery which will soon become a reality.

Parents of the future who set out to produce the perfect genetically engineered child will ultimately face a lot of disappointment, due to not accounting for the interaction of genes with each other, with their cellular environment and the inter-action of the resulting human with his or her environment. The recent film *Gattaca* presents a possible vision of the future where technology allows the selection of genetically superior traits for all offspring. The genetically superior are the privileged in this future society but there are still some 'degenerates', people whose parents have perversely not availed of the opportunity to select the best genes and have left it to chance. At one point such humans are referred to as God-children. These people are of in-ferior status and are given menial jobs. The central theme in *Gattaca* is how some of those designed to be genetically superior fail and some of those so-called degenerates can succeed – the genetic determinism is inevitably incomplete. Sixty years before *Gattaca*, Huxley presented a similar vision in *Brave New World* where the naturally born children were the 'savages' and out-casts (Huxley, *Brave New World*).

We have no reason to doubt that genetic engineering will have appeal to parents in our competitive, consumer society. There are examples galore of the lengths parents will go to gain competitive advantage for their children. What we see before us is simply a new means to that end. We have already many exam-ples of parental efforts to select the best possible offspring which is, for all intents and purposes, a private form of eugenics. In 1980, the Californian millionaire Robert Graham started a sperm bank with donors who were Nobel Prize winners. He had plenty of interested potential parents but the project collapsed because he could only interest two Nobel Prize winners, both of whom were in their 70s, and customers weren't too keen on the idea of elderly sperm, however illustrious the provenance. So he changed to employing gifted young men with some success. Abortion of damaged or simply unwanted offspring is another form of eugenics that is already widely practised.

At the moment geneticists are also looking for genes associated with high IQ, alcoholism, and homosexuality. Are we facing a future where parents will be able to decide not to carry to term a foetus carrying genes associated with homosexuality? Or can eliminate that genes or genes with who knows what consequences for their offspring's personality and pattern of interests and achievements? From what we know at the moment it is very unlikely that there is just one gene which inevitably determines homosexuality so one is talking about, at most, a level of predisposition. There are, it seems to me, extraordinary implications for the human race if we are to permit tampering with genes with the goal of preventing the birth of possibly gay or lesbian people. That will never happen, you may say, but in fact whether it will happen or not depends crucially upon how such differences are seen by a society at any point in time. Homosexuality was among the attributes that condemned many to death fifty-five years ago in the death camps in Nazi Germany. We see in attitudes to homosexuality similar processes to those which are obtained in our attitudes to disability or any condition that is seen as troublesome or undesirable.

Geneticists, arguing for the wonderful benefits which their science will bring, emphasise the potential impact of their discoveries on those who are suffering from heart-rendingly serious hereditary conditions. But hand in hand with the technologies that allow such medical interventions comes the knowledge that permits interventions that are for social, not medical, reasons. This is a feature of scientific advance. The splitting of the atom opened the door to both cheap domestic electricity for millions and the atom bomb and Chernobyl.

Looking at the vista before us, it is clear why commentators on genetic and reproductive technology are expressing concerns about the commodification of human beings. Parents, they fear, will order designer babies as someone orders a new car, specifying its colour, horsepower, the fabric to be used in its upholstery. Archbishop Desmond Connell raised this issue in his recent controversial address in Maynooth when he said, 'The child produced by the decisions of the parents begins to look more and more like a technological product. This is clear in the case of *in vitro* fertilisation, surrogate motherhood, genetic engineering, and cloning, but it may not be altogether absent in the practice of family planning.' (Connell, *The Irish Times*) Most of the Archbishop's speech focused on contraception and he did not elaborate on his concerns about the newer forms of reproductive technology, but he was right to draw attention to the slippery slope we are already standing on. Many of us would insist on our right to control the number and timing of our children and can point to the advantages this confers on us and our children in contrast to leaving it to chance or nature or God. But where will our insistence on choice lead us when we are given the kind of powers that genetics seems to promise? What values will guide our choices and how will we know the long-term consequences of our usually short term, self-interested decision-making? We may, for apparently good reasons, choose to eliminate genes carrying disease and find that genes or gene was needed in a subtle way that we had failed to understand. The example available to us now is sickle cell anaemia. If children inherit the recessive gene from both parents they will inherit this distressing condition, but carrying one gene confers resistance to malaria. As the poet Emerson said when he defined a weed: 'a weed is a plant whose virtues have not yet been discovered'. When we enter the realm of gene enhancement the dangers are even more apparent. The whims of fashion and prejudice may prevail. What appear to us today as unfortunate defects may offer advantages in the future. And what we define today as defects tomorrow we might recognise as interesting and valuable. Meanwhile a gene may have been eliminated from a family or from a society.

And is there a danger that children will come to be seen as products or commodities, not as loved and special little individuals with their own unpredictable assortment of talents and foibles, strengths and weaknesses. Parents of children born by IVF have rightly protested that they love their children and value them totally for who they are. But if in the future a couple paid a quarter of a million pounds for a genetically gifted child and she turned out to be just average, how would they view that child?

So many issues arise, many of which cannot be touched upon in a short paper. Unless people generally become aware of the issues and debate them and make informed decisions through the normal political and legislative channels, the potential for misuse of these powerful technologies will indeed be profound. The debate has begun in Ireland, but it is not very widespread. So far, action has centred on genetically modified food and our discussions about reproductive technology keep on circling around the vexed topic of abortion. It is time to broaden the debate.

Unfortunately, there are barriers that are in the way of societal engagement with these issues. The first may be our capacity to habituate and adjust. Our flexibility and capacity to take change on board, social and technological change is enormous, so that what would once have seemed alien quickly becomes normal. The second may be our willingness to leave it to the scientists. In his recent book, *Brave New Worlds*, Appleyard says there is a danger that people will sleep through this moment. They will slip into that most risky of modern habits – leaving science to the scientists. The third may be a definite difficulty for non-geneticists and members of the public in understanding what is going on. For many people science is something they stopped thinking about when they finished Junior Certificate or its equivalent. The subject matter of genetics is complex and the language technical. Nonetheless, there are scientists and science who make a very good effort at explaining its intricacies to lay people and we should be attending to what they say, just as scientists should be listening to the insights brought to them by philosophers, theologians, social scientists, and the man and woman in the street. We cannot afford a communication divide.

At this time we are brought face to face with very fundamental ontological issues. What kind of being are we and what do we value about ourselves? Do we debate and critically examine our values or do we let it all just happen? In 1946 when he wrote the foreword to the second edition of *Brave New World* which he had written in 1931, Aldous Huxley comments that 'the theme of

Brave New World is not the advancement of science as such: it is the advancement of science as it affects human individuals. The really revolutionary revolution is to be achieved not in the external world but in the souls and flesh of human beings.' The revolution is here. The question is, are we ready for it?

Notes

CHAPTER THREE

1. *Chambers Dictionary*, Chambers Harrap, Edinburgh, 1993.
2. *Wordsworth Dictionary of Biography*, Helicon Publishing, Ware (Herts), 1994.
3. Boyd, K. M., Higgs, R., and Pinching, A.J., *The New Dictionary of Medical Ethics*, British Medical Journal Publishing Group, London, 1997, p. 120.
4. American Holistic Nurses' Association, 'AHNA Philosophy', *Journal of Holistic Nursing*, 10/4,1992, p. 367.
5. Wilson, M., *Health is for People*, Darton, Longman and Todd, London, 1975.
6. Tschudin, V., *Ethics in Nursing; The Caring Relationship*, Heinemann, London, 1986, p. viii.
7. Thomasset, A., 'Narrativity and Hermeneutics in Professional Ethics', *Ethical Perspectives*, 3/4, 168-174, 1996, p. 169.
8. Taels, J., 'Ethics and Subjectivity', *Ethical Perspectives*, 2/4, 1995, p. 170.
9. Taels, J., 'Ethics and Subjectivity', *Ethical Perspectives*, 2/4, 1995, p. 170.
10. Taels, J., 'Ethics and Subjectivity', *Ethical Perspectives*, 2/4, 1995, p. 167.
11. Taels, J., 'Ethics and Subjectivity', *Ethical Perspectives*, 2/4, 1995, p. 170.
12. Rogers, C.R., *A Way of Being*, Houghton Mifflin Co., Boston, 1980, pp. 115-117.
13. Schultz, L., 'Not for resuscitation: two decades of challenge for nursing ethics and practice', *Nursing Ethics*, 4/3, 1997, pp. 227-238.
14. Thomasset, A., 'Narrativity and Hermeneutics in Professional Ethics', *Ethical Perspectives*, 3/4, 168-174, 1996, p. 169.
15. van Hooft, S., 'The Meanings of Suffering', *Hastings Centre Report*, 28/5, 1998, pp. 13-19.
16. Zohar, D., and Marshall, I., *The Quantum Society; Mind, Physics and a New Social Vision*, HarperCollins, London, 1994.

CHAPTER FOUR

Bibliography:

Arndt, M., *Ethik Denken – Masstäbe zum Handeln in der Pflege*, Georg Thieme Verlag, Stuttgart, 1996.

Finnis, J. and Fisher, A., 'The Four Principles and Their Use' in R. Gillon, ed., *Principles of Healthcare Ethics*, John Wiley & Sons, Chichester: New York, 1994, pp. 31-44.

Government of the Republic of Ireland, *Report of The Commission on Nursing – A Blueprint for the Future*, Government Publications, Dublin, 1998.

Harris, J., *The Value of Life*, Routledge & Kegan Paul, London, 1985.

Hart, G., 'College-based Education: Background and Bugs', *The Australian Nurses Journal*, 15(4), pp. 46-48 in *Report of The Commission on Nursing – A Blueprint for the Future*, Government Publications, Dublin, 1998.

Horster, D., *Habermas zur Einführung*, Junius Verlag, Hamburg, 1990.

Hunt, G., 'Abortion: Why Bioethics Have No Answer', *Nursing Ethics*, 6 (1), 1999, pp. 47-57.

Köchli, D.I., *Ein heisses Eisen*, Die Weltwoche, Zürich, 1999, p. 23.

Küng, H., *Global responsibility*, London: SCM Press, London, 1990.

Minogue, B., *Bioethics – A Committee Approach*, Jones and Bartlett Publishers, Boston, London, 1996.

Rowe, C., 'Ethics in Ancient Greece' in P. Singer, ed., *A Companion to Ethics*, Basil Blackwell Ltd, Oxford, 1993, pp. 121-131.

Seedhouse, D., *Ethics – The Heart of Healthcare*, John Wiley & Sons, Chichester, New York, 1988.

Singleton, J. and McLaren, S., *Ethical Foundations of Healthcare*, Mosby, London, 1995.

Veatch, *A Theory of Medical Ethics*, Basic Books, New York, 1981.

Williams, A., 'Economics, Society and Healthcare ethics' in R. Gillon, ed., *Principles of Healthcare Ethics*, John Wiley & Sons, Chichester: New York, 1994, pp. 829-842.

World Health Organisation, *Constitution*, WHO, Geneva, 1948.

World Health Organisation, *Health for All in the 21st century*, WHO, Geneva, 1998.

Yach, D., 'Health and Illness: The Definition of the World Health Organisation' *Ethik in der Medizin*, 10 (Supplement), 1998, pp. 7-13.

CHAPTER SIX

1. Shepherd, M., 'Foreword to General Psychopathology' in Shepherd, M. and Zagrill, O.L., eds., *Handbook of Psychiatry*, Vol. 1, Cambridge University Press, Cambridge, 1983, p. ix.

2. Lewis, A., 'Health as a Social Concept', *British Journal of Sociology*, 4, 1953, pp. 109-24.

3. World Health Organisation, *The ICD-10 Classification of Mental and Behavioural Disorders*, World Health Organisation, Geneva, 1992.

4. American Psychiatric Association, *DSM-IV, Diagnostic and Statistical Manual of Mental Disorders*, American Psychiatric Association, Washington, 1994.

5. Block, S. and Chodoff, P., 'Introduction', in Block, S. and Chodoff, P., eds., *Psychiatric Ethics*, Oxford Medical Publications, Oxford University Press, Oxford, 1991, p. l.

6. Norman, C., 'Family Care of Persons of Unsound Mind', *Transactions of the Conference of Irish District Asylums*, November, 1903.

7. Department of Health, *Green Paper on Mental Health*, The Government Stationery Office, Dublin, 1992.

8. Block, S. and Chodoff, P., 'Introduction' in Block, S. and Chodoff, P., eds., *Psychiatric Ethics*, Oxford Medical Publications, Oxford University Press, Oxford, 1991.

9. Council of Europe, *The European Convention on Human Rights*, Strasbourg, 1953.

10. The Medical Council, *A Guide to Ethical Conduct and Behaviour*, 5th Edition, Dublin, 1998.

11. Department of Health, *Mental Treatment Act, 1945*, The Government Stationery Office, Dublin, 1945.

12. Szasz, T.S., *The Myth of Mental Illness*, 2nd Edition, Harper and Row, New York, 1974.

13. Peay, J., 'Bounewood: An Indefensible Gap in Mental Health Law', *British Medical Journal*, 317, 1998, pp. 94-5.

14. Tomkin, D. and McAuley A., 'Competence to Refuse Medical Intervention', *Medicine Weekly*, 9 December, 38, 1998.

15. Stone, A.A., 'Psychiatric Abuse and Legal Reform' in Stone, A.A., ed., *Law, Psychiatry and Morality*, American Psychiatric Press, Inc., Washington, 1984, pp. 133-160.

16. Gutheil, T.G., 'In Search of True Freedom: Drug Refusal, Involuntary Medication and rotting with your rights on', *American Journal of Psychiatry*, 137, 1980, pp. 577-80.

17. Phillips, M., 'Forget psychiatry, stop psychopaths', *The Sunday Times*, October 25th, 1998.

18. Editorial, 'Straw's judgement: a delicate balance between liberty and society', *The Sunday Times*, February 22nd, 1999.

19. Ramsay, 'UK Psychiatrists Refuse to Treat the Untreatable' *Lancet*, 353, 647, 1999.

20. Szasz, T., *Cruel Compassion: Psychiatric Control of Society's Unwanted*, John Wiley & Sons, Inc., Chichester: New York, 1994.

CHAPTER SEVEN

Cases Cited:
Attorney-General v X [1992] 1 I. R. 1
McGee v Attorney-General [1974] IR, 284
In Re Conroy 486 A. 2d 1209 [1985]
In Re Jobes 529 A. 2d 434 [1987]
In Re Peter 529 A. 2d 419 [1987]
Re A Ward of Court [1995] 2 ILRM. 401
Re R (Adult: Medical Treatment) [1996] 2 FLR 99

Bibliography:
Bataille, Georges, *Eroticism* (trans. Dalwood, M.), Marion Boyars, London, 1987.

Beck, Ulrich, *Risk Society: Towards A New Modernity*, Sage, London, 1992.

Berkovitch, Nitza, 'Motherhood as a National Mission: The Construction of Womanhood in the Legal Discourse in Israel', *Women's Studies International Forum*, Volume 20, 1997, pp. 606-19.

British Medical Association, *Advance Statements about Medical Treatment: Code of Practice*, BMA, London, 1995.

British Medical Association, *Withdrawing and Withholding Treatment: A Consultation Paper from the BMA's Medical Ethics Committee*, BMA, London, 1998.

British Medical Association and Royal College of Nursing, *Decisions Relating to Cardiopulmonary Resuscitation: A Statement from the BMA and the RCN in association with the Resuscitation Council*, 1993.

Callahan, Daniel, *The Troubled Dream of Life: Living with Mortality*, Simon and Schuster, New York, 1993.

Costello, Rose, 'Supreme Court decision "a clear case of euthanasia"', *The Cork Examiner*, 28 July, 1995, p. 4.

Dworkin, Ronald, *Life's Dominion: An Argument About Euthanasia and Abortion*, HarperCollins, London, 1993.

Dworkin, Ronald, 'Assisted Suicide: The Philosopher's Brief', *The New York Review of Books*, XLIV, 1997, pp. 41-2.

Frank, Arthur, *The Wounded Storyteller: Body, Illness and Ethics*, University of Chicago Press, Chicago, 1995.

Giddens, Anthony, *Modernity and Self-Identity: Self and Society in the Late Modern Age*, Polity Press, Cambridge, 1991.

Harmon, D., 'Falling off the Vine: Legal Fictions and the Doctrine of Substituted Judgement', *Yale Law Journal*, Volume 110, Number 1, 1990, pp. 1-71.

Irish Medical Council, *A Guide to Ethical Conduct and to Fitness to Practise*, The Medical Council, Dublin, 1994.

Irish Medical Council, *Statement of the Council after their statutory meeting on 4th August, 1995*, The Medical Council, Dublin, 1995.

Irish Medical Council, *A Guide to Ethical Conduct and Behaviour*, The Medical Council, Dublin, 1998.

Irish Nursing Board, 'Guidance of the Irish Nursing Board of 18th August, 1995', The Nursing Board, Dublin, 1995.

Lipovetsky, Gilles, *Le Crepescule du Devoir*, Gallimard, Paris, 1991.

Lord Chancellor's Department, *Who Decides? Making Decisions on Behalf of Mentally Incapacitated Adults*, The Stationery Office, London, 1997.

Meisel, Alan, *The Right to Die*, John Wiley and Sons, Chichester: New York, 1989.

Minow, Martha, *Making All the Difference: Inclusion, Exclusion and American Law*, Cornell University Press, Ithaca, 1990.

Murphy-Lawless, Jo and McCarthy, James, 'Social Policy and Fertility Change in Ireland: The Push to Legislate in Favour of Women's Agency', *The European Journal of Women's Studies*, Volume 6, 1999, pp. 69-96.

O'Mahony, Patrick and Delanty, Gerard, *Rethinking Irish History: Nationalism, Identity and Ideology*, Macmillan, Basingstoke, 1998.

O'Toole, F. 'Archbishop's insensitivity arises from ignorance', *Irish Times*, March 5, 1999, p. 8.

Pabst Battin, Margaret, *The Least Worst Death: Essays in Bioethics on the End of Life*, Oxford University Press, New York, 1994.

Ricks, Christopher, *Beckett's Dying Words*, Oxford University Press, New York, 1995.

Shilling, Chris, *The Body and Social Theory*, Sage, London, 1993.

Smyth, Ailbhe, '"And Nobody was any the Wiser": Irish Abortion Rights and the European Union', in R. A. Elman, ed., *Sexual Politics and the European Union*, Berghahn, Providence, Rhode Island, 1996, pp. 109-30.

Sunstein, Cass, 'The Right to Die', *The Yale Law Journal* Volume 106, Number 4, 1997, pp. 1123-64.

Sunstein, Cass, *One Case at a Time: Judicial Minimalism on the Supreme Court*, Harvard University Press, Cambridge, 1999.

Teff, Harvey, *Reasonable Care: Legal Perspectives on the Doctor-Patient Relationship*, Clarendon Press, Oxford, 1994.

Waldby, Catherine, *AIDS and the Body Politic: Biomedicine and Sexual Difference*, Routledge, London, 1996.

CHAPTER EIGHT

Bibliography:

Appleyard, B., *Brave New Worlds: Genetics and the Human Experience*, HarperCollins, London, 1999.

Bronfenbrenner, U., *The Ecology of Human Development*, Harvard University Press, Cambridge, 1979.

Connell, D., 'Child resents a parentage based on power', *The Irish Times*, Monday, March 18, 1999.

Dawkins, R., 2nd ed., *The Selfish Gene*, Oxford University Press, Oxford, 1989.

Dennett, D., 'Conditions of Personhood' in M. F. Goodman, *What is a Person?*, Human Press, Clifton, NJ, 1988.

Doran, K., *What is a Person? The Concept and the Implications for Ethics*, Edwin Mellen Press, Lampeter, 1989.

Greene, S., 'What Makes a Person a Person? The Limits and Limitations of Genetics' in M. Junker-Kenny, ed., *Designing Life? Genetics, Procreation and Ethics*, Ashgate, London, 1999.

Goodman, M. F., *What is a Person?*, Human Press, Clifton, NJ, 1988.

Gourevich, P., *We Wish to Inform You that Tomorrow We Will Be Killed With Our Families: Stories from Rwanda*, Picador, London, 1999.

Haraway, D.J., *Simians, Cyborgs and Women*, Free Association Books, London, 1999.

Hubbard, R., 'Abortion and Disability: Who Should and Who Should

Not Inhabit the World?' in L.J. Davis, *The Disability Studies Reader*, Routledge, London, 1997.

Huxley, A., *Brave New World*, Flamingo, London, 1946/1994.

Kurzweil, R., *The Age of Spiritual Machines: When Computers Exceed Human Intelligence*, Viking Penguin, New York, 1999.

Marteau, T. and Richards, M., *The Troubled Helix: Social and Psychological Implications of the New Genetics*, Cambridge University Press, Cambridge, 1995.

Norton, A., 'Why There is No Concept of a Person', in C. Gill, ed., *The Person and the Human Mind*, Clarendon Press, Oxford, 1990.

Pinker, S., *How the Mind Works*, Penguin, Harmondsworth, 1994.

Rich, A., 2nd ed., *Of Woman Born*, W. W. Norton, London, 1986.

Silver L., *Remaking Eden: Cloning and Beyond in a Brave New World*, Wiedenfeld and Nicolson, London, 1998.

Wilmut, I., Schnieke, A.E., McWhir, J., Knid, A.J. and Campbell, K.H.S., 'Viable Offspring Derived from Fetal and Adult Mammalian Cells', *Nature*, 385, 810-13, 1997.